CARDIOVASCULAR IMAGING REVIEW

CARDIOVASCULAR IMAGING REVIEW

Nancy K. Koster, MD
Assistant Professor of Medicine
Division of Cardiology
Creighton University School of Medicine
Omaha, Nebraska

ELSEVIER
SAUNDERS

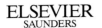

1600 John F. Kennedy Blvd.
Ste. 1800
Philadelphia, PA 19103-2899

CARDIOVASCULAR IMAGING REVIEW   ISBN: 978-1-4160-6250-9

Notice

Knowledge and best practice in this field are constantly changing. As new research and experience broaden our understanding, changes in research methods, professional practices, or medical treatment may become necessary.

Practitioners and researchers must always rely on their own experience and knowledge in evaluating and using any information, methods, compounds, or experiments described herein. In using such information or methods they should be mindful of their own safety and the safety of others, including parties for whom they have a professional responsibility.

With respect to any drug or pharmaceutical products identified, readers are advised to check the most current information provided (i) on procedures featured or (ii) by the manufacturer of each product to be administered, to verify the recommended dose or formula, the method and duration of administration, and contraindications. It is the responsibility of practitioners, relying on their own experience and knowledge of their patients, to make diagnoses, to determine dosages and the best treatment for each individual patient, and to take all appropriate safety precautions.

To the fullest extent of the law, neither the Publisher nor the authors, contributors, or editors, assume any liability for any injury and/or damage to persons or property as a matter of products liability, negligence or otherwise, or from any use or operation of any methods, products, instructions, or ideas contained in the material herein.

Library of Congress Cataloging-in-Publication Data
Koster, Nancy K.
  Cardiovascular imaging review / Nancy K. Koster. — 1st ed.
      p. ; cm.
  Includes bibliographical references and index.
  ISBN 978-1-4160-6250-9 (pbk. : alk. paper)
  1. Cardiovascular system—Magnetic resonance imaging—Atlases. 2. Cardiovascular system—
Diseases—Diagnosis—Magnetic resonance imaging—Atlases. I. Title.
  [DNLM: 1. Cardiovascular Diseases—diagnosis—Atlases. 2. Diagnostic Imaging—Atlases. WG 17]
  RC670.5.M33K67 2011
  616.1'07548—dc22   2011011939

Executive Publisher: Natasha Andjelkovic
Developmental Editor: Brad McIlwain
Publishing Services Manager: Pat Joiner-Myers
Senior Project Manager: Joy Moore
Design Direction: Steven Stave

Printed in China.

Last digit is the print number: 9 8 7 6 5 4 3 2 1

I would like to dedicate this book to my husband, Mike, my three daughters, Emily, Lindsey, and Kaylie, and to all the cardiovascular fellows of Creighton University School of Medicine.

CONTRIBUTORS

Bradley Davis, RT(R)(CV)(CT)(ARRT)
Cardiac Catheterization Laboratory
Creighton University Medical Center
Omaha, Nebraska
Angiography

Michael G. Delcore, MD, FACC
Associate Professor of Medicine
Division of Cardiology
Creighton University School of Medicine
Omaha, Nebraska
Angiography

Scott E. Fletcher, MD, FAAP, FACC, FSCAI
Professor of Pediatrics
Joint Division of Pediatric Cardiology
University of Nebraska/Creighton University
Children's Hospital and Medical Center
Omaha, Nebraska
Cardiovascular Magnetic Resonance Imaging

M. Jeff Holmberg, MD, PhD, FACC, FASE
Associate Professor of Medicine
Division of Cardiology
Creighton University School of Medicine
Omaha, Nebraska
Echocardiography

Kim Jenkins, ARRT(R)(MR)
Oklahoma Heart Institute
Tulsa, Oklahoma
Cardiovascular Magnetic Resonance Imaging

Alan Kaneshige, MD, FACC, FASE
AHS Oklahoma Heart Institute
Tulsa, Oklahoma
Cardiovascular Magnetic Resonance Imaging

Olaf Kaufman, MD, PhD
Cardiovascular/Interventional Radiology
Methodist Hospital, Iowa Radiology
Des Moines, Iowa
Cardiovascular Computed Tomography

Jacob S. Koruth, MD
Cardiovascular Fellow
Division of Cardiology
Creighton University School of Medicine
Omaha, Nebraska
Electrocardiography

Nancy K. Koster, MD
Assistant Professor of Medicine
Division of Cardiology
Creighton University School of Medicine
Omaha, Nebraska
*Electrocardiography; Echocardiography;
Questions and Answers*

Shelby Kutty, MD, FACC, FASE
Assistant Professor of Pediatrics
Joint Division of Pediatric Cardiology
University of Nebraska/Creighton University
Children's Hospital and Medical Center
Omaha, Nebraska
Cardiovascular Magnetic Resonance Imaging

Thomas J. Lanspa, MD, FASA
Associate Professor of Medicine
Division of Cardiology
Creighton University School of Medicine
Omaha, Nebraska
Angiography

Edward T. Martin, MD, FACC, FACP, FAHA
Director, Cardiovascular MRI
Oklahoma Heart Institute
Tulsa, Oklahoma
Cardiovascular Magnetic Resonance Imaging

Vicki Moore, ARRT(N)(R), CNMT
Oklahoma Heart Institute
Tulsa, Oklahoma
Cardiovascular Magnetic Resonance Imaging

Aryan N. Mooss, MD, FACC
Professor of Medicine
Division of Cardiology
Creighton University School of Medicine
Omaha, Nebraska
Electrocardiography

Ann E. Narmi, MD
Cardiovascular Fellow
Division of Cardiology
Creighton University School of Medicine
Omaha, Nebraska
Angiography

Julie Ratino, MD
Radiology Resident
Division of Radiology
Creighton University School of Medicine
Omaha, Nebraska
Cardiovascular Computed Tomography

Susan M. Schima, MD
Assistant Professor of Medicine
Division of Cardiology
Creighton University School of Medicine
Omaha, Nebraska
Questions and Answers

John W. Sype, MD, FACC, FSCAI
The Everett Clinic Heart and Vascular
    Department
Everett, Washington
Angiography

Senthil Thambidorai, MD
Cardiovascular Fellow
Division of Cardiology
Creighton University School of Medicine
Omaha, Nebraska
Electrocardiography

Michael D. White, MD
Assistant Professor of Medicine
Division of Cardiology
Creighton University School of Medicine
Omaha, Nebraska
Angiography

Special thanks to Nathan Dix of the Creighton
    University IT Department for his technical
    expertise.

PREFACE

This cardiovascular imaging resource is geared toward physicians, physicians in training, and other medical professionals interested in gaining knowledge of or reviewing cardiovascular disease and pathology through imaging and electrocardiography. This book is complemented by a companion Expert Consult website containing fully searchable text, images, and questions. Using imagery, this print and online resource can help solidify a physician's or trainee's knowledge of the vast array of cardiovascular diseases and pathology. In addition, this book lends itself to a quick-but-comprehensive "look through" to glean clinical pearls in preparation for certification or recertification examinations in Internal Medicine or Cardiovascular Diseases.

Electrocardiography continues to be of prime importance in the investigation and diagnosis of various cardiovascular diseases. Chapter 1 is an extensive compilation of common and interesting electrocardiograms often seen in clinical practice. Chapters 2 to 5 contain echocardiograms, angiograms, cardiovascular CTs, and cardiovascular MR images of both common and rarely encountered diseases. After studying the included images, the reader's knowledge of the cardiovascular system and the diseases affecting it should be more easily recalled. Finally, 100 multiple-choice, board-style questions are provided at the end of the book. These questions address topics commonly encountered during the American Board of Internal Medicine Cardiovascular and Internal Medicine examinations. Succinct explanations and references are included with the answers.

The adage "a picture is worth a thousand words" was the impetus and inspiration for this book. Although it is necessary for physicians and trainees to comprehensively study the pathology and diseases that affect the cardiovascular system, visualization of the diseases and pathology enables one to more quickly comprehend and recall the information. I hope readers find this book to be an interesting and useful resource during their study and review of cardiovascular diseases and during preparation for certification or recertification examinations.

Nancy K. Koster, MD
Omaha, Nebraska

CONTENTS

GLOSSARY

2D	two-dimensional
3D	three-dimensional
AAA	abdominal aortic aneurysm
ACC	American College of Cardiology
ACE	angiotensin-converting enzyme
AHA	American Heart Association
AMI	anterior myocardial infarction
AP	anteroposterior
ARB	angiotensin receptor blocker
ASD	atrial septal defect
AV	atrioventricular
AVM	arteriovenous malformation
AVNRT	atrioventricular nodal reentry tachycardia
AVRT	atrioventricular reentrant tachycardia
b.i.d.	twice a day
BP	blood pressure
bpm	beats per minute
BSA	body-surface area
BUN	blood urea nitrogen
CABG	coronary artery bypass graft
CAD	coronary artery disease
CBC	complete blood count
CHF	congestive heart failure
CNS	central nervous system
COPD	chronic obstructive pulmonary disease
Cr	creatinine
CT	computed tomography
DDDR	dual-chamber rate-adaptive pacemaker
DHA	docosahexaenoic acid
DVT	deep vein thrombosis
ECA	external carotid artery
ECG	electrocardiogram
EEG	electroencephalography
EMB	endomyocardial biopsy
EOA	effective orifice area
EPA	eicosapentaenoic acid
EPS	electrophysiologic study
FFP	fresh frozen plasma
GCM	giant cell myocarditis
GI	gastrointestinal
Hb	hemoglobin
HbA$_{1c}$	glycosylated hemoglobin
HCM	hypertrophic cardiomyopathy
HDL	high-density lipoprotein
IABP	intra-aortic balloon pump
IART	intra-atrial reentrant tachycardia
ICA	internal carotid artery
ICD	implantable cardioverter defibrillator
ICP	intracranial pressure
INR	International Normalized Ratio
I.M.	intramuscular
I.V.	intravenous
IVC	inferior vena cava
IVCD	interventricular conduction delay
K	potassium
LAD	left anterior descending artery

LAD	left axis deviation
LAE	left atrial enlargement
LAO	left anterior oblique
LAFB	left anterior fascicular block
LBBB	left bundle branch block
LCA	left coronary artery
LCX	left circumflex artery
LDL	low-density lipoprotein
LICS	left intercostal space
LIMA	left internal mammary artery
LMCA	left main coronary artery
LV	left ventricle
LVH	left ventricular hypertrophy
LVOT	left ventricular outflow tract
MCA	middle cerebral artery
MI	myocardial infarction
MIP	maximal intensity projection
MRA	magnetic resonance angiography
MRI	magnetic resonance imaging
Na	sodium
NHLBI	National Heart, Lung and Blood Institute
NSAID	nonsteroidal anti-inflammatory drug
NSTEMI	non-ST elevation myocardial infarction
NSVT	nonsustained ventricular tachycardia
NYHA	New York Heart Association
PA	pulmonary artery
PAC	premature atrial contraction
PAPVR	partial anomalous pulmonary venous return
PCI	percutaneous intervention
PCP	primary care provider
PCWP	pulmonary capillary wedge pressure
PDA	patent ductus arteriosus
PDA	posterior descending artery
PLA	posterior lateral artery
PMI	point of maximal impulse
PMT	pacemaker-mediated tachycardia
PPM	prosthesis–patient mismatch
PVC	premature ventricular contraction
PVD	peripheral vascular disease
RAD	right axis deviation
RAE	right atrial enlargement
RAO	right anterior oblique
RBBB	right bundle branch block
RCA	right coronary artery
RUPV	right upper pulmonary vein
RV	right ventricle
RVH	right ventricular hypertrophy
RVOT	right ventricular outflow tract
SAH	subarachnoid hemorrhage
SAM	systolic anterior motion of the mitral valve
SFA	superficial femoral artery
STEMI	ST-segment elevation myocardial infarction
SVC	superior vena cava

SVG	saphenous vein graft	**TV**	tricuspid valve
SVT	supraventricular tachycardia	**UFH**	unfractionated heparin
TC	total cholesterol	**VLDL**	very low-density lipoprotein
TEE	transesophageal echocardiogram	**Vo$_2$**	oxygen consumption
TGA	transposition of the great arteries	**VSD**	ventricular septal defect
TIA	transient ischemic attack	**VT**	ventricular tachycardia
t.i.d.	three times a day	**VVI**	ventricular demand inhibited
TPA	tissue plasminogen activator		pacemaker
TSH	thyroid-stimulating hormone	**WB**	white blood
TTE	transthoracic echocardiogram	**WPW**	Wolff-Parkinson-White

CARDIOVASCULAR IMAGING REVIEW

ELECTROCARDIOGRAPHY

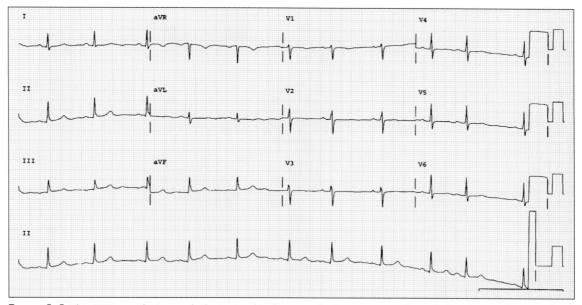

FIGURE 1-1 This ECG reveals sinus arrhythmia. For this diagnosis the P-wave axis and morphology have to be normal with a gradual change in the P-P interval. The difference between the shortest and longest P-P intervals must be >10%.

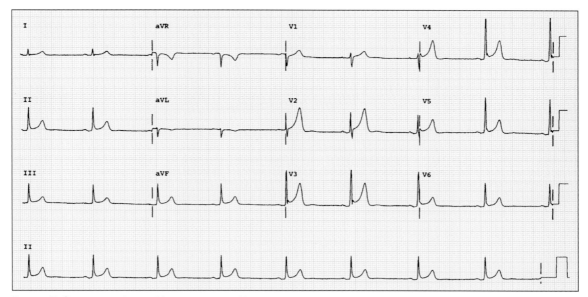

FIGURE 1-2 An ECG obtained from a 28-year-old male college basketball player. It displays sinus bradycardia with early repolarization (normal variant).

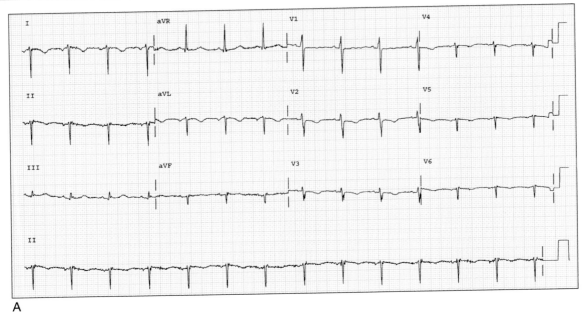

A

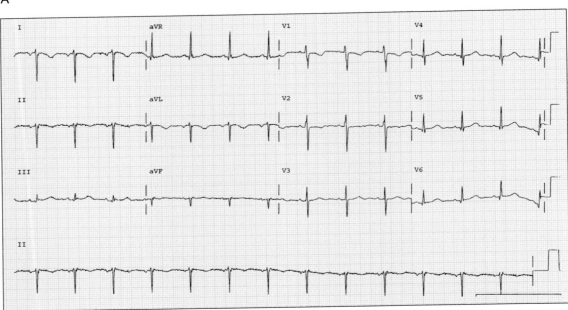

B

FIGURE 1-3 A, This ECG was obtained on a routine physical examination in a 50-year-old male. The ECG displays sinus rhythm and findings consistent with dextrocardia. Note the positive P waves and upright QRS in lead aV_R and the reverse in leads I and aV_L. Also note that the R-wave progression in the chest leads is reversed. **B,** A subsequent ECG was obtained for this patient. In this ECG the chest leads are rearranged onto the right precordium, correcting the abnormal R-wave progression. If the above information was not known, one would then comment on left and right arm lead reversal in their interpretation.

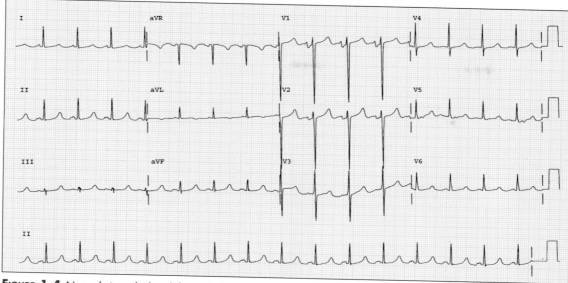

FIGURE 1-4 Normal sinus rhythm, left atrial abnormality, LVH, and prolonged QT interval (487 ms). The criteria for LAE include a notched P wave with duration ≥ 0.12 s in inferior leads (P mitrale) and terminal downward deflection of the P wave in V_1 with negative amplitude of 1 mm and duration of 0.04 ms.

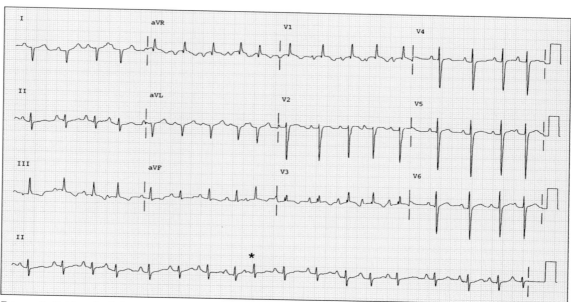

FIGURE 1-5 Note the following findings on this ECG: normal sinus rhythm, sinus arrhythmia, RAD, LAE, RAE, RVH with ST-segment and/or T-wave abnormality secondary to hypertrophy. Lead V_2 and V_3 are reversed. Finally, an atrial premature complex is present (*asterisk*).

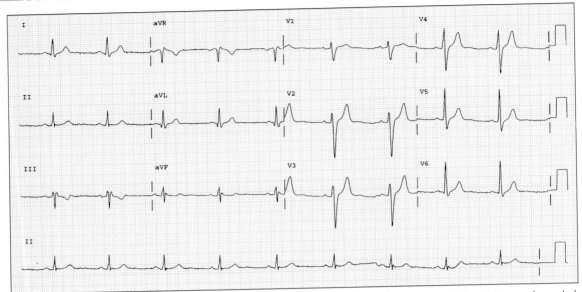

FIGURE 1-6 This ECG reveals sinus rhythm with a nonspecific IVCD. The criteria for IVCD are QRS ≥ 110 ms and morphology not meeting criteria for either LBBB or RBBB. Some of the common causes include conduction system disease, antiarrhythmic drug toxicity, hyperkalemia, WPW syndrome, and hypothermia.

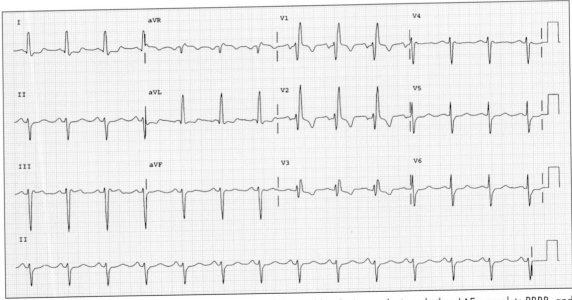

FIGURE 1-7 This ECG was obtained in an asymptomatic 84-year-old male. It reveals sinus rhythm, LAE, complete RBBB, and LAFB. Criteria for LAFB include frontal plane axis of −45° to −90°, qR pattern in lead aV$_L$, R peak time in lead aV$_L$ of 45 msec or more, and QRS duration less than 120 msec in absence of a RBBB.

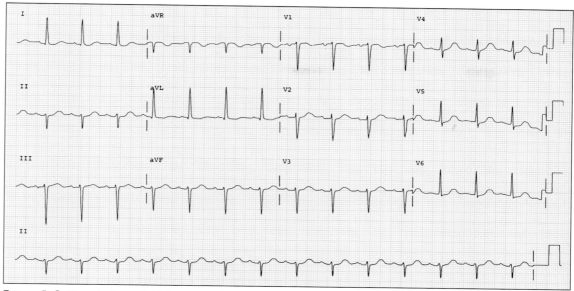

FIGURE 1-8 Sinus rhythm with LAFB. Criteria for LAFB are axis between −45° and −90°, qR complex in lead aV$_L$, R peak time in lead aV$_L$ of 45 msec or more, and QRS duration less than 120 msec. In addition, other reasons for LAD such as LVH or inferior infarct should be absent. Remember in the presence of LAFB, voltage criteria for LVH using the R-wave amplitude in lead aV$_L$ in isolation is not applicable.

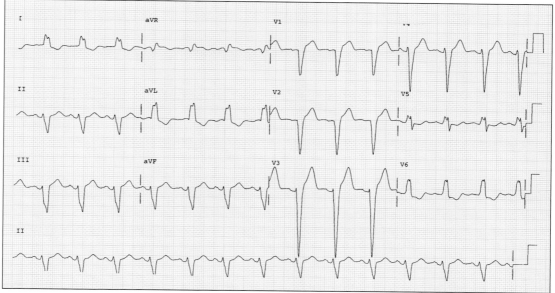

FIGURE 1-9 This ECG was obtained in a 65-year-old female with cardiomyopathy. It demonstrates sinus rhythm and complete LBBB. For a diagnosis of complete LBBB the following criteria should be present: QRS duration > 120 ms; delayed intrinsicoid deflection in the left-sided precordial leads (V$_5$ and V$_6$); broad monophasic R waves in leads I, aV$_L$, V$_5$, and V$_6$; QS or rS complex in lead V$_1$; and absent septal Q waves in the left-sided leads.

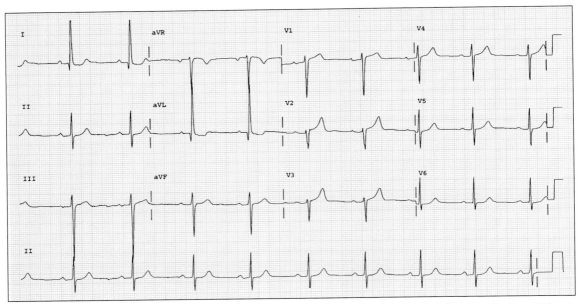

FIGURE 1-10 A 34-year-old male with exertional shortness of breath. The ECG reveals sinus bradycardia (rate 50 bpm), voltage criteria for LVH with pseudo Q waves in leads I and aV_L. An echocardiogram confirmed the diagnosis of HCM.

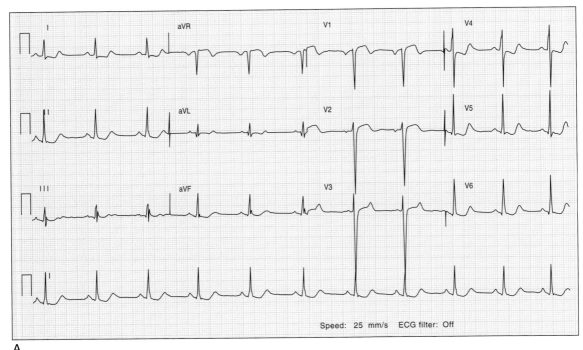

A

FIGURE 1-11 A, This ECG was obtained in a 29-year-old male with a history of HCM with a significant outflow tract gradient of 90 mm Hg. The ECG reveals sinus rhythm, LAE, and LVH with ST-T abnormalities due to hypertrophy.

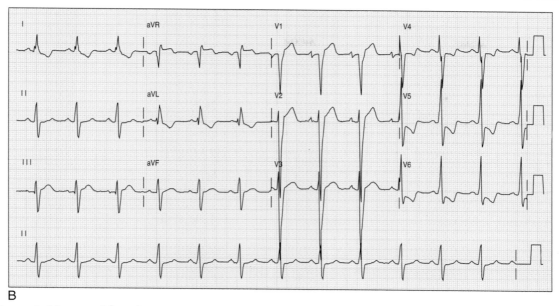

B

FIGURE 1-11—cont'd B, The same patient, after failing medical therapy, underwent surgical septal resection. Postoperatively he developed an IVCD resembling LBBB.

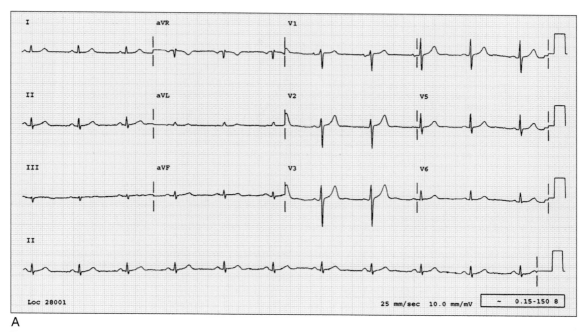

A

FIGURE 1-12 A, A 56-year-old male presented to the emergency department promptly after the onset of precordial chest pain, nausea, and shortness of breath. An ECG was obtained that revealed normal sinus rhythm with low voltage in the frontal leads.

Continued

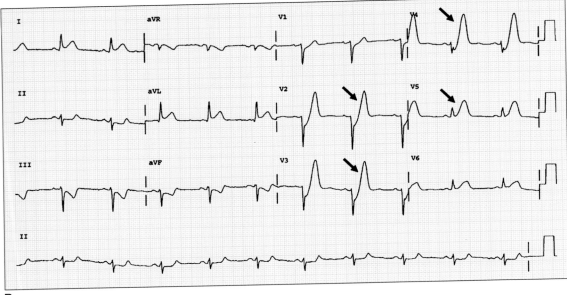

B

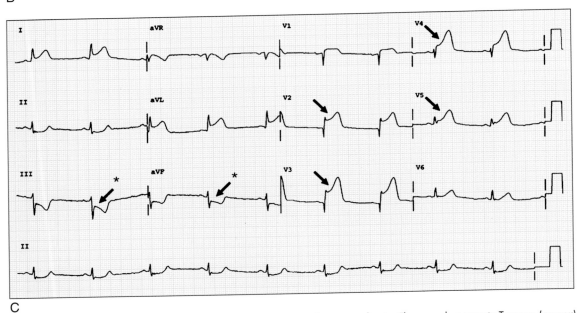

C

FIGURE 1-12—cont'd B, This ECG was obtained 30 minutes after onset of pain. There are hyperacute T waves (*arrows*) in the precordial leads, suggesting acute anterolateral myocardial injury. ST-segment elevation is present in leads I and aV$_L$. Reciprocal changes of ST-segment depression and T-wave inversion are noted inferiorly. **C,** A third ECG was obtained as the patient was being prepared for the cardiac catheterization laboratory. ST-segment elevation (*arrows*) and anterior Q waves developed indicative of acute anterior and lateral MI/injury. Note reciprocal ST-segment depression (*arrows with asterisks*) in the inferior leads.

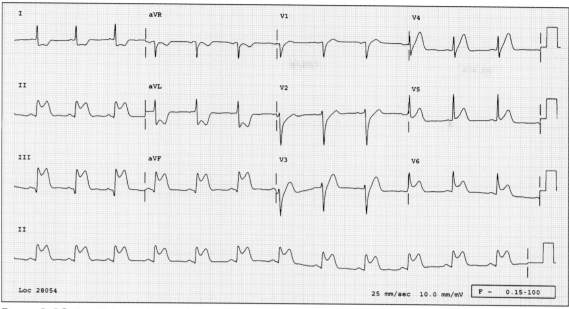

FIGURE 1-13 This ECG reveals sinus rhythm with acute inferolateral injury. ST-segment elevation is present in leads II, III, aV$_F$, V$_5$, and V$_6$. Reciprocal ST-segment depression is present in the high lateral leads, I and aV$_L$. Diagnostic Q waves consistent with acute inferior infarction are present in lead III but borderline in aV$_F$.

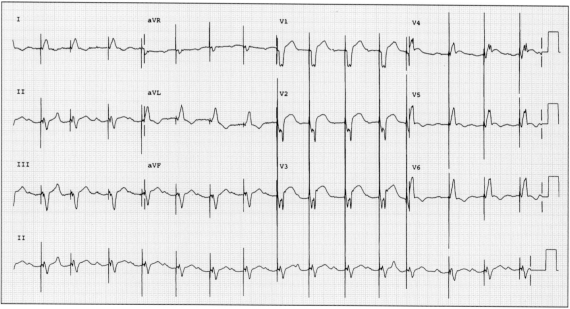

FIGURE 1-14 This ECG reveals sinus rhythm, first-degree AV block, and an atrial-sensed and ventricular-paced rhythm. An acute AMI is evident on this ECG. Note the primary ST-segment and T-wave changes best seen in V$_4$ and V$_5$.

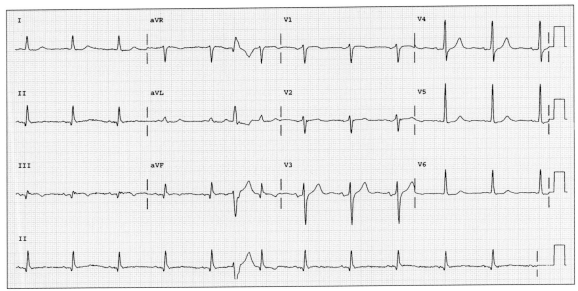

FIGURE 1-15 This ECG reveals sinus rhythm with an interpolated PVC and an age-indeterminate inferior wall MI. An interpolated PVC occurs most often when the sinus rate is slow and it does not disturb the sinus rhythm.

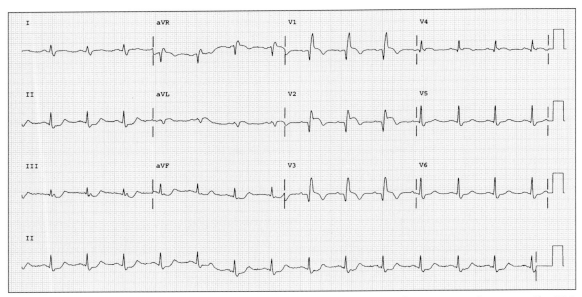

FIGURE 1-16 This 69-year-old male presented with sudden onset of chest pain to the emergency department. The ECG reveals sinus rhythm, RBBB, with Q waves and ST-segment elevation in leads V_1 to V_4, suggesting acute anteroseptal STEMI. Note RBBB does not interfere with the diagnosis of AMI as LBBB does.

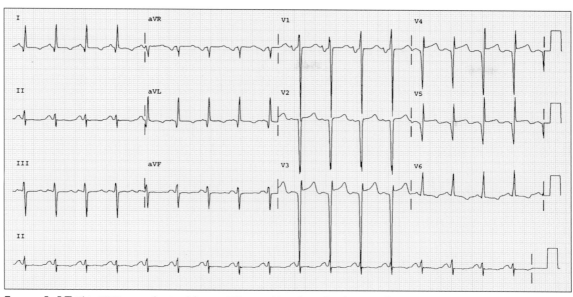

FIGURE 1-17 This ECG was obtained from a 78-year-old male with a history of MI 10 years ago. He is followed in a heart failure clinic. The ECG reveals normal sinus rhythm, LAE, borderline LAD, and an old anterior and lateral MI. There is persistent ST-segment elevation anteriorly, suggesting ventricular aneurysm.

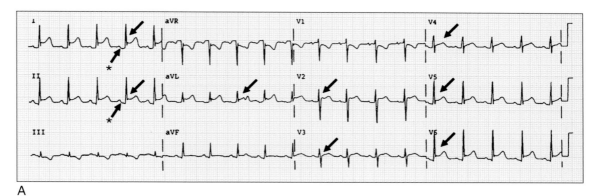

FIGURE 1-18 A, An ECG of a 43-year-old male who presented with fevers, body aches, and chest pain on inspiration reveals sinus rhythm, diffuse ST-segment elevations (*arrows*) (except in leads aV$_R$ and V$_1$), and PR-segment depression (*arrows with asterisks*), best visualized in leads I and II. These changes suggest acute pericarditis. Other findings that may be present in such cases are tachycardia, low-voltage QRS complexes, and electrical alternans. **B,** Follow-up ECG of the same patient demonstrates typical evolutionary changes in acute pericarditis. Interval resolution of the ST-segment elevation and inversion of T waves are now present.

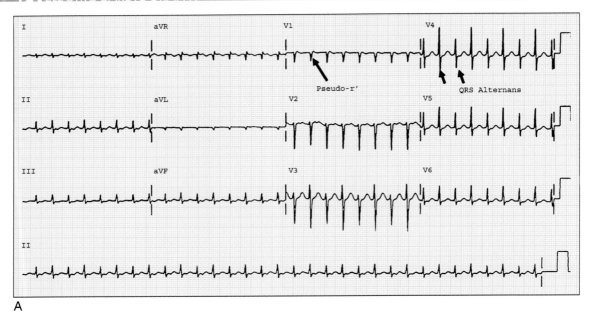

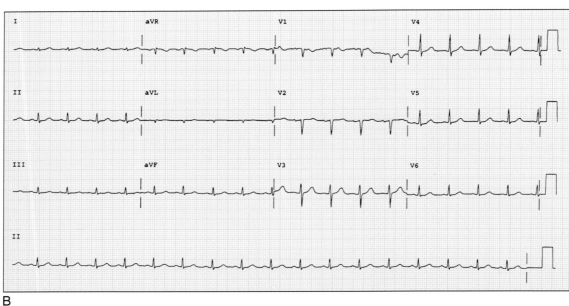

FIGURE 1-19 A, An ECG of a 32-year-old male who presented with sudden onset of palpitations reveals a narrow complex tachycardia (SVT). Note the pseudo-r′ (retrograde P wave; *long arrow*) seen in the terminal portion of lead V₁, suggesting AVNRT. QRS alternans (*short arrows*), noted here, is often present during SVT. **B,** The patient received I.V. adenosine, which terminated his SVT, and this ECG was then obtained. Findings indicate normal sinus rhythm. Note the normal appearance of the QRS complex in lead V₁. Compare this with the morphology in lead V₁ during the tachycardia.

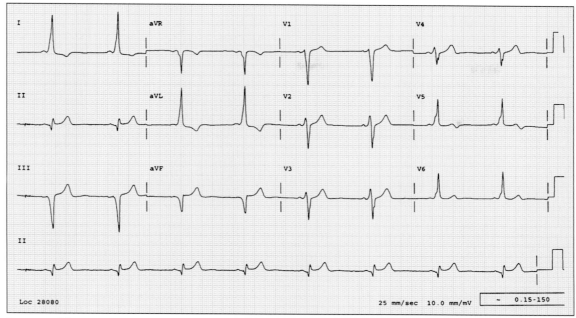

FIGURE 1-20 This 54-year-old male presented to his PCP with a history of palpitations. The ECG reveals sinus bradycardia, short PR interval, delta waves (positive and best seen in leads I, aV$_L$, V$_5$, and V$_6$), suggesting ventricular preexcitation (WPW syndrome). There are negative delta waves inferiorly, simulating inferior Q waves. Electrocardiographically this suggests a right posteroseptal accessory pathway. There are ST-T wave changes in leads I, aV$_L$, and V$_5$ that are due to repolarization abnormalities.

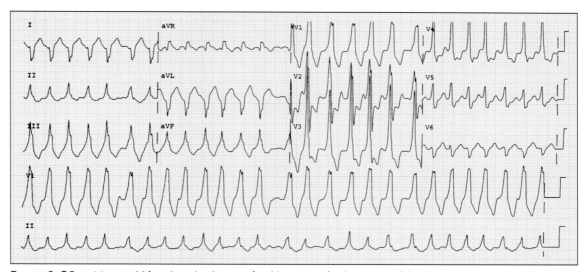

FIGURE 1-21 A 28-year-old female with a history of sudden onset of palpitation and dizziness that required cardioversion. The ECG reveals a rapid irregular wide complex tachycardia. This is atrial fibrillation with rapid ventricular response, with the variable conduction defects seen due to underlying preexcitation (WPW syndrome). A diagnosis of MI, axis deviation, or ventricular hypertrophy should not be made when underlying preexcitation is present.

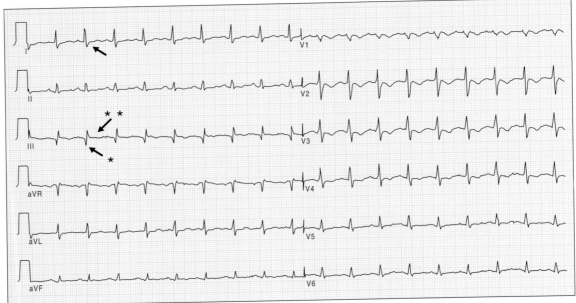

Figure 1-22 This ECG was obtained from a patient presenting with syncope and hypoxia. Sinus tachycardia with S1Q3T3 pattern (S1, *arrow*; Q3, *arrow with asterisk*; T3, *arrow with double asterisks*) is present, suggestive of pulmonary embolism. Anterior T-wave inversions in this case are consistent with right ventricular strain. In the appropriate clinical setting, such as in this case, the ECG findings are consistent with the diagnosis of acute cor pulmonale from a pulmonary embolus.

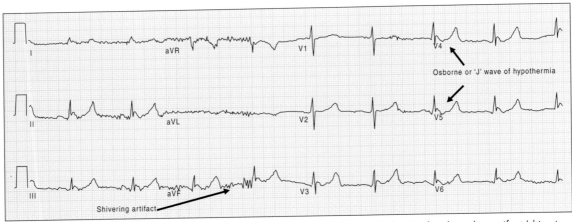

Figure 1-23 This ECG was obtained in a patient with hypothermia. Findings include sinus bradycardia, artifact (shivering; *long arrow*), prolonged QT interval, and J waves/Osborne waves (*short arrows*).

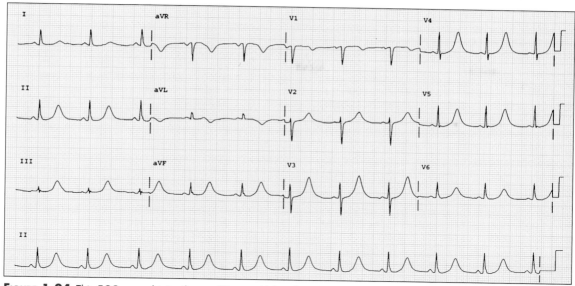

FIGURE 1-24 This ECG was obtained on a 39-year-old female with meningitis and altered mental status. It reveals sinus rhythm and prolonged QT interval secondary to acute CNS injury. Tall T waves may also suggest hyperkalemia but are often narrow-based unlike these wide-based T waves. Other changes that may be present in a patient with CNS injury include deeply inverted T waves, prominent U waves, ST-segment elevation or depression, and multiple rhythm abnormalities.

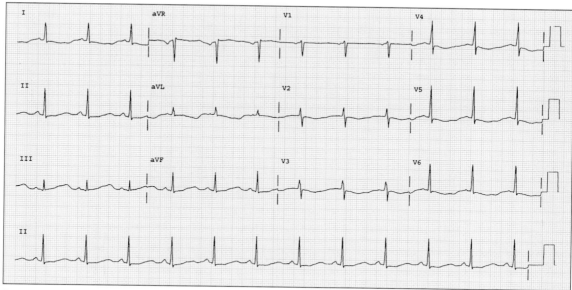

FIGURE 1-25 This ECG was obtained on an unresponsive patient after the patient underwent cardioversion for polymorphic VT. Her potassium level was 2.2 mEq/L. The ECG shows sinus rhythm with marked QT prolongation and ST-T abnormalities secondary to hypokalemia.

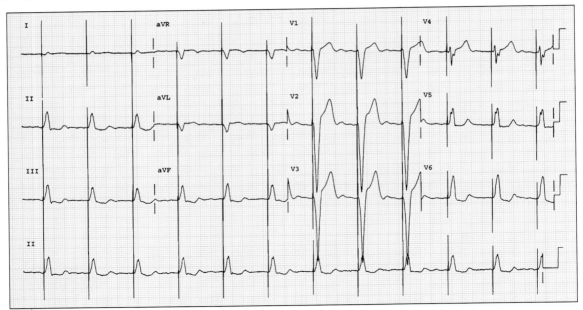

FIGURE 1-26 Ventricular-paced rhythm with underlying atrial fibrillation. Note the absence of underlying P waves, suggesting underlying atrial fibrillation. This ECG was obtained from a 70-year-old male with a history of symptomatic bradycardia and chronic atrial fibrillation who received a single-chamber ventricular pacemaker.

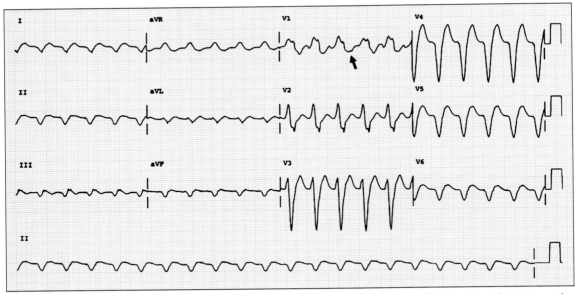

FIGURE 1-27 A 58-year-old male with a history of ischemic cardiomyopathy presents with a regular wide QRS complex tachycardia (125 bpm) with an indeterminate axis consistent with VT. Findings favoring ventricular origin include QRS morphology resembling a RBBB with R > r′, QRS width > 140 ms, and the time from the beginning of R wave to nadir of s wave > 100 ms. The deflection seen in lead V_1 is suggestive of AV dissociation (*arrow*).

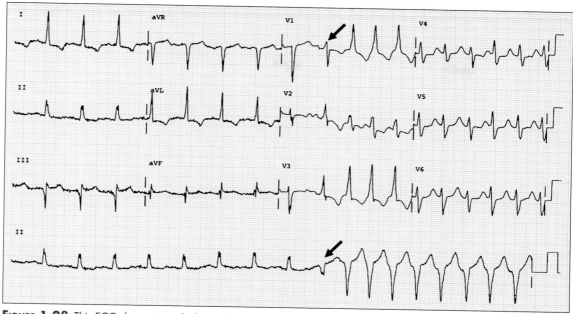

FIGURE 1-28 This ECG shows sinus rhythm with LVH with ST-T wave abnormalities due to hypertrophy. The second half of the ECG reveals VT with a fusion beat (*arrow*) at the onset. The presence of a fusion beat is evidence of AV dissociation, and a monophasic R wave in V_1 is also consistent with VT.

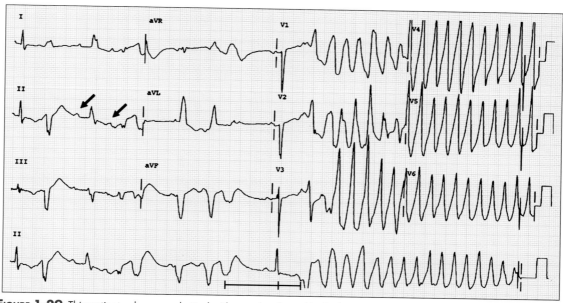

FIGURE 1-29 This patient, who was admitted with complete heart block, then developed bradycardia-induced polymorphic VT (ventricular rates, 250 bpm). This ECG shows the atria and ventricle to be dissociated in the initial half of the tracing (note P waves marked with the *arrows*). There are multiform PVCs present. In the middle of the tracing there is a sinus beat normally conducted, followed by a fusion beat and then the onset of polymorphic VT. Note the long–short sequence (marked in the figure with *brackets*), which often occurs before the onset of this arrhythmia.

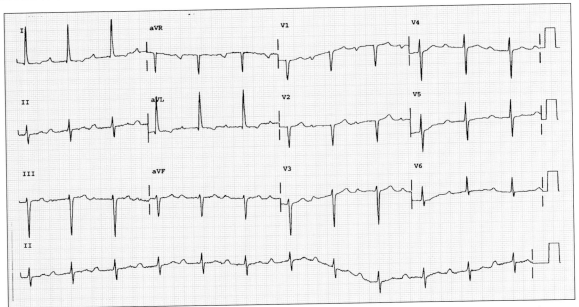

FIGURE 1-30 This ECG reveals sinus rhythm with first-degree AV block, LAE, and LVH with secondary ST/T wave changes.

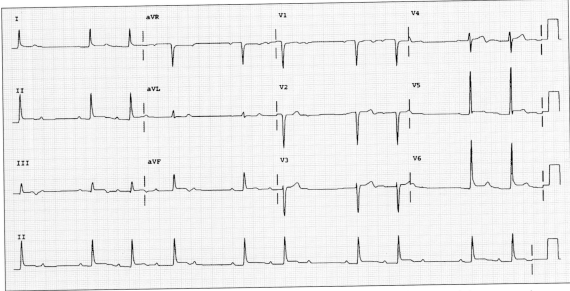

FIGURE 1-31 This 52-year-old male was seen in the emergency department with sudden onset of chest pain and nausea. The ECG reveals sinus rhythm and LVH by voltage criteria. There are subtle ST-T wave abnormalities, suggesting injury, in the inferior and lateral leads. Finally, second-degree Mobitz type I AV block (Wenckebach) is present. Note when the shortest PR interval following the Wenckebach sequence has a PR interval > 200 ms, first-degree AV block is also present. Criteria for Mobitz type I AV block are progressive PR prolongation, then block; progressive RR shortening, then block; RR interval containing nonconducted P wave < 2 P-P intervals; and group beating.

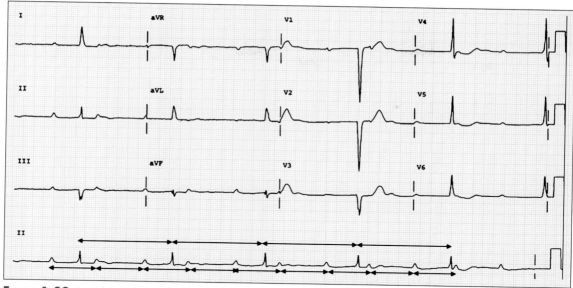

FIGURE 1-32 An 84-year-old male presented to the emergency department with presyncopal spells on exertion. The ECG revealed complete heart block with a junctional escape rhythm at a rate of 34 bpm. Note the dissociation of the P waves and QRS complexes. There is voltage criteria for LVH with secondary ST-T wave changes and an incomplete LBBB (QRS = 118 ms).

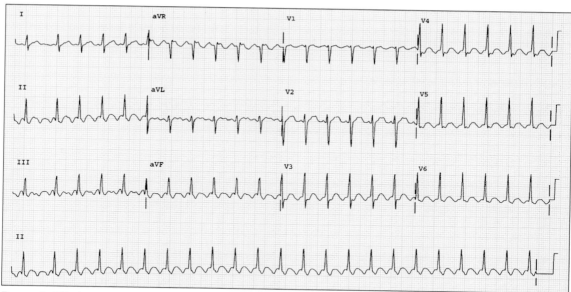

FIGURE 1-33 This ECG reveals atrial flutter with 2:1 AV block. This can often be difficult to diagnose. The clue lies in the heart rate close to 150 bpm. Flutter waves are usually at rates of 240–340 bpm as opposed to atrial tachycardia with atrial rates < 240 bpm.

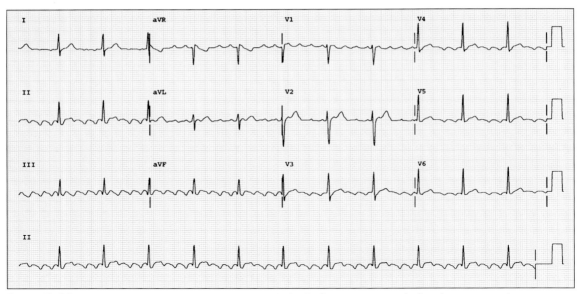

FIGURE 1-34 This ECG reveals atrial flutter with 4:1 AV block. The flutter waves give the baseline a saw-tooth appearance, which is best seen in the inferior leads.

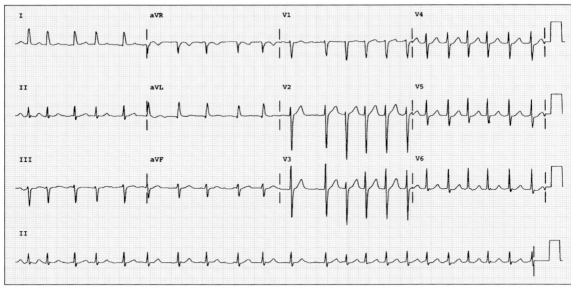

FIGURE 1-35 This ECG demonstrates atrial fibrillation with rapid ventricular response. Note that P waves are absent, and there is irregularity of the R-R intervals.

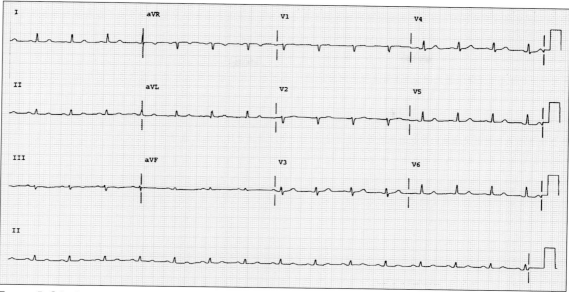

FIGURE 1-36 This ECG reveals low voltage in both limb (R+S < 5 mm) and precordial (R+S < 10 mm) leads. Depending on the accompanying clinical situation, consider the following common diagnoses: pericardial effusion, COPD, and myxedema. Other causes, such as morbid obesity and infiltrative myocardial diseases, are also possibilities.

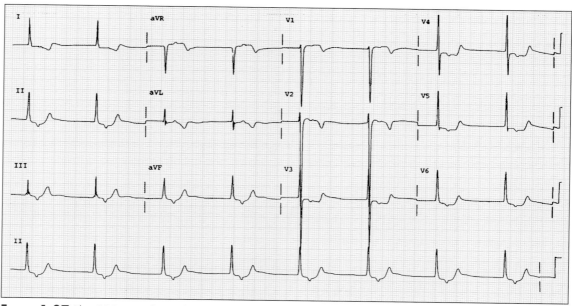

FIGURE 1-37 This ECG was obtained in an 80-year-old lethargic male. The rhythm is junctional bradycardia with retrograde P waves (note the inverted P waves in the inferior leads). Other findings include LVH with secondary ST-T wave changes.

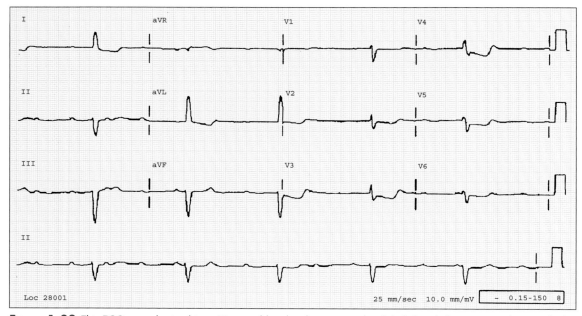

FIGURE 1-38 This ECG was obtained in a 60-year-old male who presented with light-headedness. It reveals sinus rhythm at a rate of 88 bpm with complete heart block and a ventricular escape rhythm at a rate of 34 bpm.

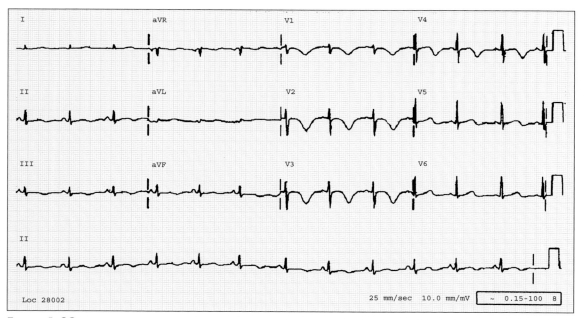

FIGURE 1-39 A 60-year-old female presented to the emergency department with chest pain. Coronary angiography revealed normal coronary arteries. Her ECG is characteristic of apical ballooning syndrome, also known as Takotsubo cardiomyopathy. Sinus rhythm with diffuse broad-based T-wave inversions and prolongation of the QT interval (600 ms) is present. Differential diagnosis would include CNS pathology, apical variant of HCM, pheochromocytoma, myocarditis, and anterior ischemia. In apical ballooning syndrome, ST-segment elevation may be the initial ECG finding at the time of presentation during active chest pain.

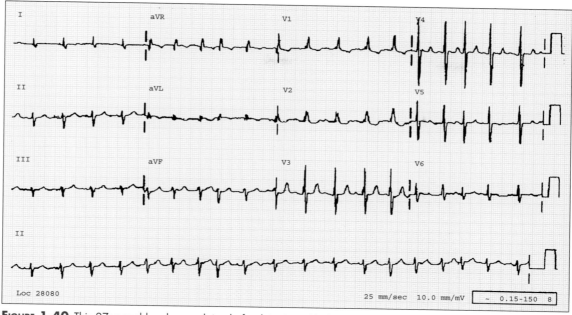

Loc 28080   25 mm/sec   10.0 mm/mV   ~ 0.15-150   8

FIGURE 1-40 This 27-year-old male complained of palpitations. His ECG revealed sinus tachycardia with frequent atrial premature complexes, an incomplete RBBB, and LAD. A complete or incomplete RBBB with LAD is characteristic of an ostium primum ASD, which was diagnosed by echocardiography in this patient.

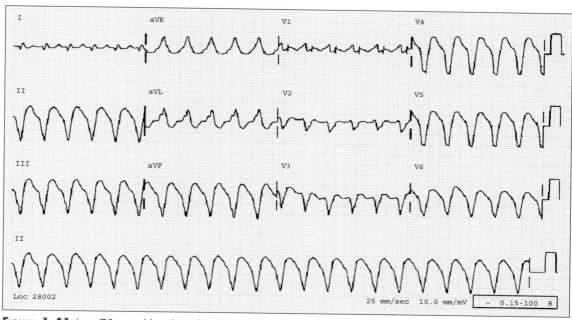

Loc 28002   25 mm/sec   10.0 mm/mV   ~ 0.15-100   8

FIGURE 1-41 In a 75-year-old male with a dual-chamber pacemaker, an ECG revealed a paced rhythm at a rate of 130 bpm, which was the upper rate limit set for his device. He was treated initially by applying a magnet over the pacemaker, which terminated this rhythm. He had PMT. The initiation of PMT involves the tracking of a retrograde P wave from a PVC and depolarization of the atrium before the next atrial-paced beat. This impulse can then trigger the pacemaker and a circuit is established, thereby generating PMT or endless-loop tachycardia. To prevent PMT, the pacemaker is programmed so the atrial lead is insensitive to the retrograde P wave. This is accomplished by increasing the post-ventricular atrial refractory period.

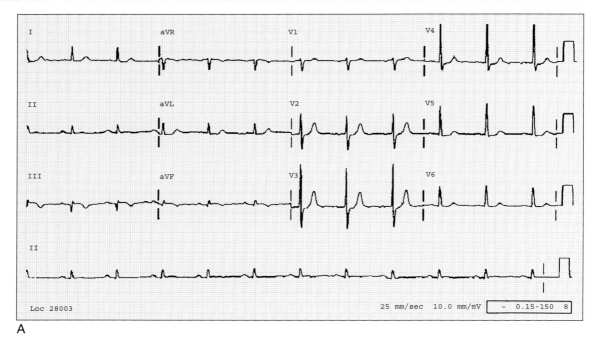

A

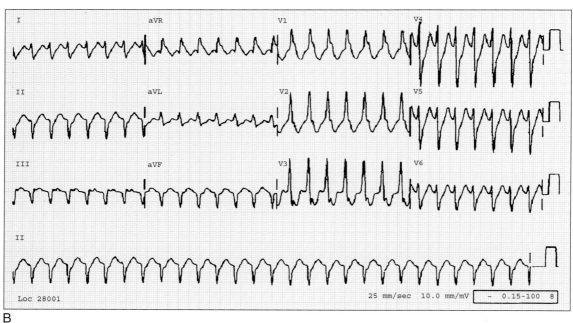

B

FIGURE 1-42 A, ECG of an 86-year-old female shows sinus rhythm and an inferior infarct, age indeterminate. She was hospitalized for evaluation of syncope. **B,** This ECG, obtained during her hospitalization, reveals a wide-complex tachycardia consistent with VT. Features suggestive of VT include RBBB with R > R′, QRS width > 140 ms, and change in axis from baseline to extreme northwest axis. Other features of VT not present here include AV dissociation, absence of RS complexes in precordial leads, R-to-S interval > 100 ms, and concordance across the precordial leads.

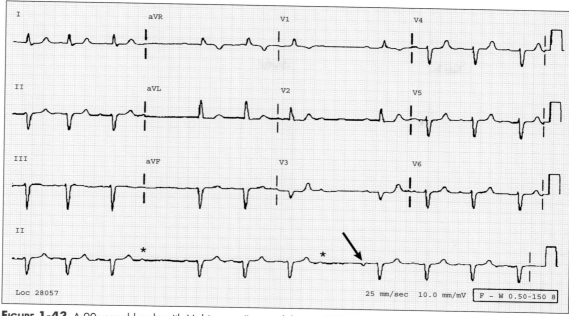

FIGURE 1-43 A 90-year-old male with Mobitz type II second-degree AV block. In type II second-degree AV block, there are intermittent blocked P waves (*asterisks*). The PR intervals of the conducted impulses are constant. However, the PR interval may be slightly shorter in the impulse following the block because of improved conduction that may occur after the blocked beat. The beat marked with an *arrow* has a slightly different P-wave morphology and is like an escape complex.

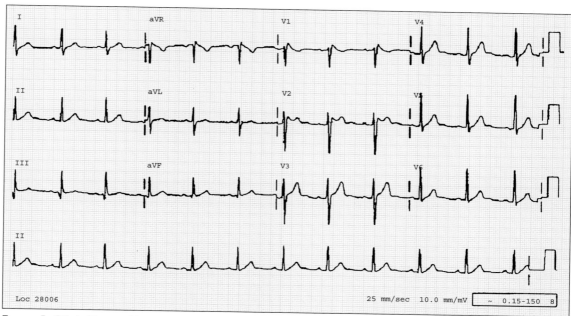

FIGURE 1-44 A 50-year-old male with Brugada ECG pattern. There is incomplete RBBB with ST-segment elevation across right precordial leads. This ECG has features of type I and type II Brugada pattern. The type I ECG pattern (noted in lead V₁) is characterized by pronounced elevation of the J point, a coved-type ST segment, and an inverted T wave. The type II pattern is characterized by ST-segment elevation >1 mm with a saddleback configuration as seen in lead V₂. The type III pattern, (not shown here), is characterized by saddleback ST-segment elevation < 1 mm.

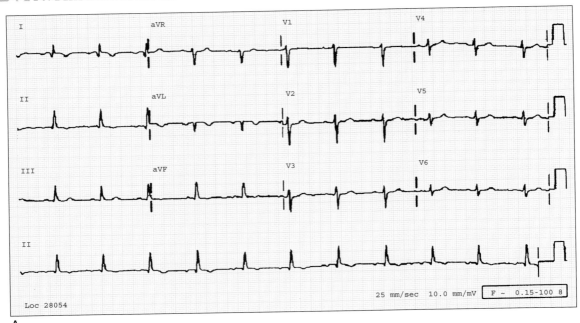

A

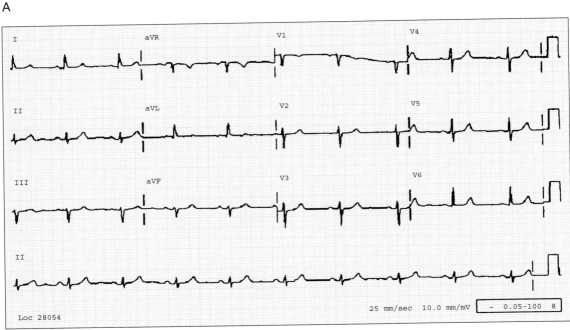

B

FIGURE 1-45 A, This ECG demonstrates limb lead reversal (left and right arm). Note the positive P wave and T wave in lead aV$_R$; negative P wave in leads I, II, and aV$_L$; and negative T wave in leads I and aV$_L$. The R-wave progression across the precordial leads is normal excluding dextrocardia. **B,** Repeat ECG after correct limb lead placement revealing normal sinus P-wave configuration and QRS and T-wave complexes.

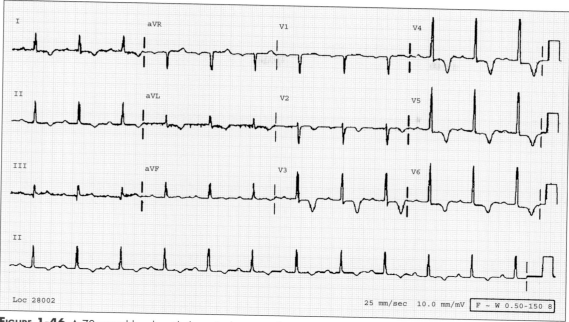

FIGURE 1-46 A 72-year-old male with the apical variant of HCM. His ECG reveals sinus rhythm with characteristic giant T-wave inversions (defined as > −10 mm in amplitude) and tall R waves across lateral precordial leads. Note first-degree AV block is present, which is also common in this variant.

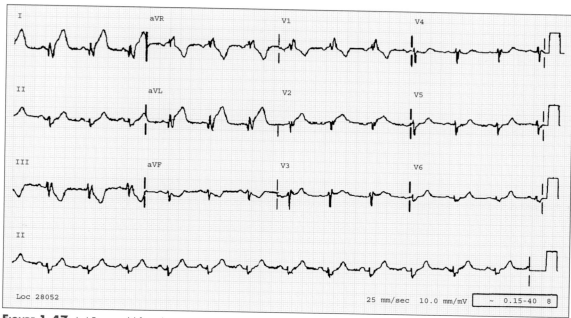

FIGURE 1-47 A 65-year-old female presenting with chest pain. ECG reveals sinus rhythm with complete RBBB. There is also ST-segment elevation in the high lateral leads (I, aV$_L$) with reciprocal ST-segment depression inferiorly. Q waves are present in leads I and aV$_L$, indicating an acute STEMI. ST-segment elevation indicative of injury can be diagnosed in RBBB, unlike in LBBB, where this finding would be masked by the bundle branch block.

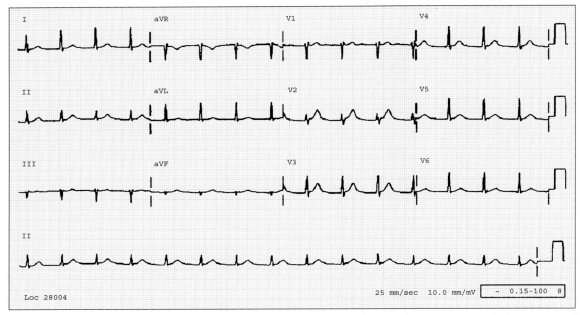

FIGURE 1-48 A 57-year-old male with digoxin overdose. His ECG revealed an accelerated junctional rhythm at a rate of 88 bpm, which is a classic rhythm seen in patients with digoxin toxicity. Paroxysmal atrial tachycardia with block is another rhythm associated with digoxin toxicity.

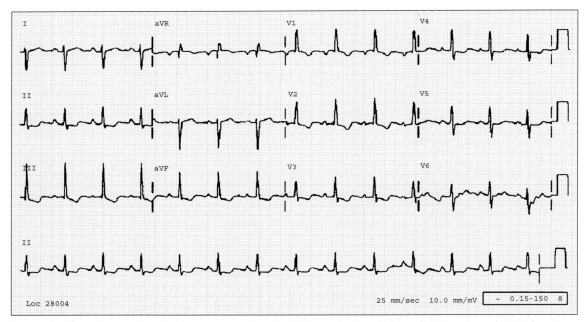

FIGURE 1-49 A 46-year-old male with shortness of breath. ECG reveals sinus rhythm with LAE, RAD, and RVH. The criteria for RVH present are: the tall R wave in lead V_1 > 6 mm, R/S ratio > 1 in lead V_1, and R/S ratio < 1 in lead V_6. A differential diagnosis for a tall R wave in lead V_1 would include posterior MI, RBBB, WPW syndrome, Duchenne muscular dystrophy, incorrect lead placement, and a normal variant.

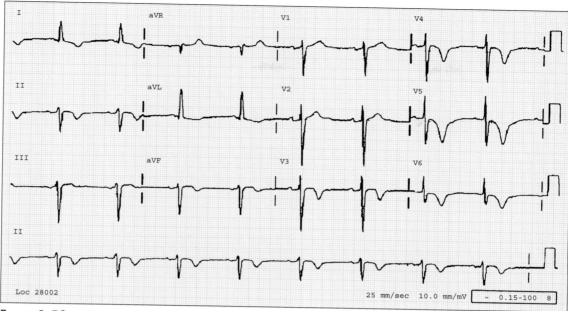

FIGURE 1-50 An 80-year-old female diagnosed with an intracranial hemorrhage. Her ECG reveals sinus rhythm with diffuse anterolateral T-wave inversions and a prolonged QT interval of 600 ms. Corrected QT interval is 547 ms. There is LAFB; hence, lead aV$_L$ cannot be used as a sole criterion for LVH.

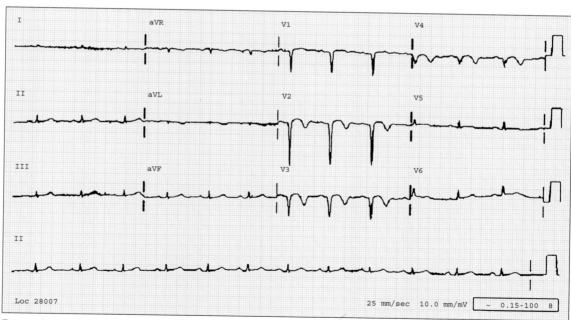

FIGURE 1-51 A 63-year-old male with a history of chest pain several weeks before admission who presented with CHF. ECG revealed sinus rhythm and a recent anterior infarct with persistent T-wave changes. Low voltage is noted in the limb leads, which is consistent with an extensive infarction.

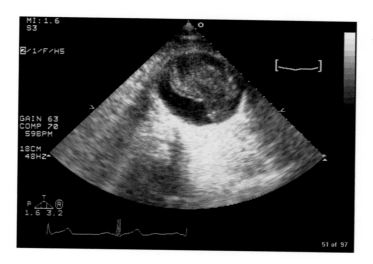

FIGURE 2-1 AAA with dissection. Thrombus fills the false lumen.

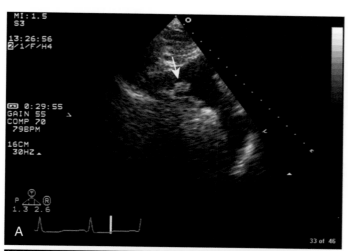

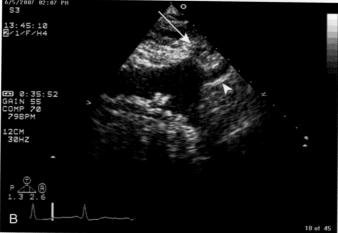

FIGURE 2-2 A, Transthoracic suprasternal notch view of the aortic arch demonstrating severe atheromatous disease of the aortic arch. The pedunculated mass (*short arrow*) is a mobile atheroma attached to the wall of the aorta by a small stalk. **B,** Similar view with the origins of the left common carotid (*long arrow*) and left subclavian (*arrowhead*) arteries noted.

FIGURE 2-3 TEE of an aortic dissection. **A,** Longitudinal view of the descending thoracic aorta. Note the intimal flap separating the true and false lumens. Color flow imaging shows blood flow within both lumens. **B,** Transverse view showing the aorta in cross-section with the intimal flap easily visualized.

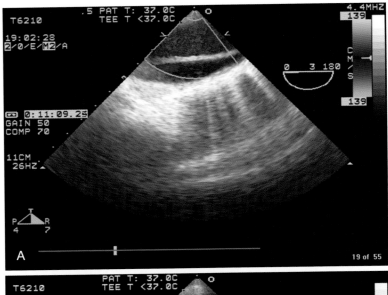

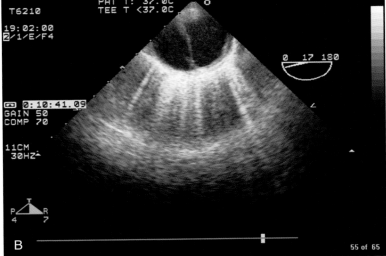

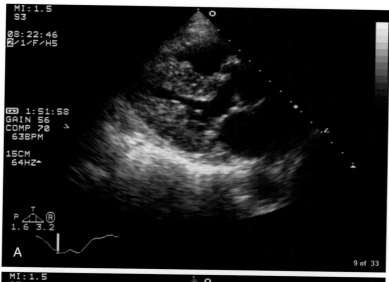

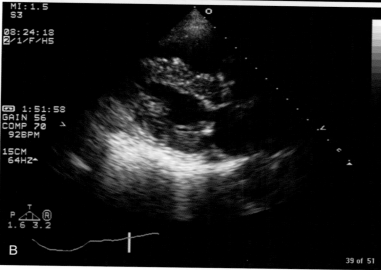

FIGURE 2-4 Parasternal long-axis view in a patient with cardiac amyloidosis. **A,** Systole. **B,** Diastole. Important findings are marked concentric LVH with granular speckled appearance of the myocardium. Generally, valve leaflets appear thickened. Although, left ventricular function is often well-preserved until late stages of the disease, diastolic dysfunction is present and is usually restrictive.

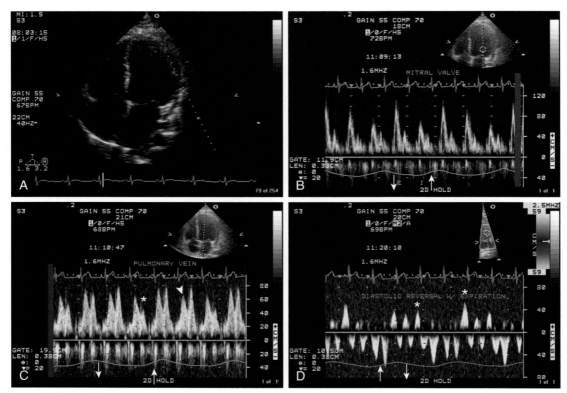

FIGURE 2-5 TEE of a 29-year-old male with recurrent constrictive pericarditis. The pericardium becomes restrictive and restrains cardiac filling. The volume within the heart nearly becomes fixed. Filling of the cardiac chambers then varies with the respiratory cycle. On inspiration, right ventricular filling increases and left ventricular filling decreases. On expiration, left ventricular filling increases and right ventricular filling decreases. This ventricular interdependence is best demonstrated using pulsed-wave Doppler. **A,** Apical four-chamber view. The left ventricular size is at the upper limits of normal. **B,** Pulsed-wave Doppler inflow of the mitral valve with simultaneous use of a respirometer (*up arrows* indicate inspiration; *down arrows* indicate expiration). With inspiration, the mitral inflow velocity decreases; with expiration, it increases. The opposite changes in filling velocities occur across the tricuspid valve. **C,** Pulmonary vein flow demonstrating that both the systolic and diastolic flow velocities decrease at the onset of inspiration (*asterisks*) and increase at the onset of expiration (*arrowhead*). **D,** With expiration, hepatic vein flow diminishes and there is significant diastolic flow reversal (*asterisks*).

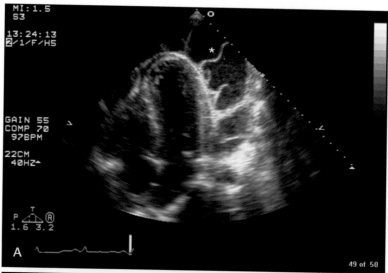

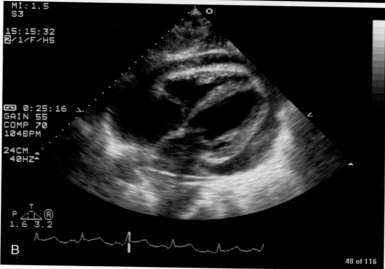

FIGURE 2-6 A, Massive pericardial effusion. Transthoracic four-chamber view of an extremely large, circumferential pericardial effusion with fibrinous stranding (*asterisk*). The right ventricular apex is compressed; note the right atrial collapse in late diastole. **B,** Subcostal view of another large circumferential pericardial effusion causing tamponade. The size and extent of a pericardial effusion is often best visualized in the subcostal view.

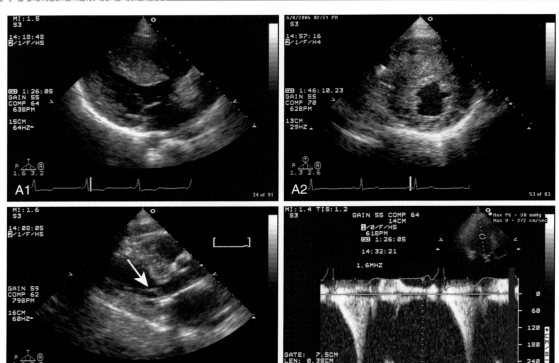

FIGURE 2-7 HCM. **A,** Parasternal long- and short-axis views demonstrating severe concentric LVH. The septum is more severely affected than the other left ventricular walls. **B,** SAM (*short arrow*) of the anterior mitral valve leaflet is a hallmark of HCM. It is best seen in the transthoracic parasternal long-axis view. **C,** Continuous wave Doppler at the level of the LVOT. Note the classic dagger-shaped pattern of flow, which peaks late in systole. The resting gradient measures 30 mm Hg. With Valsalva maneuver, the gradient often increases significantly.

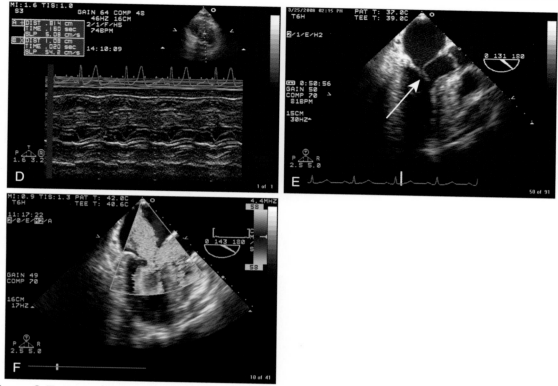

FIGURE 2-7—cont'd D, M-mode through the mitral valve displaying SAM of the anterior mitral valve leaflet. **E,** Transesophageal three-chamber view clearly showing SAM (*long arrow*) of the anterior mitral leaflet. This contributes to the dynamic obstruction of blood flow out the LVOT. **F,** Transesophageal color flow imaging showing increased velocities in the LVOT producing the *Venturi effect*, essentially pulling the anterior mitral leaflet into the outflow tract. Concurrently, mitral regurgitation occurs. In this example, the mitral regurgitation is severe.

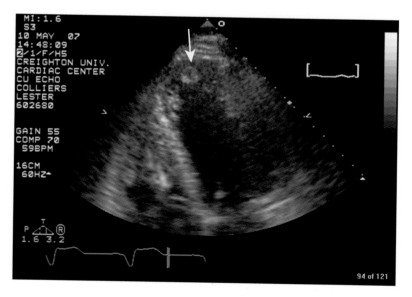

FIGURE 2-8 Transthoracic apical four-chamber view in a patient with akinesis of the apex. Note the well-circumscribed echodensity in the left ventricular apex consistent with thrombus (*arrow*).

FIGURE 2-9 A, Apical four-chamber view showing thrombi (*arrows*) in the left and right ventricular apices in a patient with idiopathic dilated cardiomyopathy. **B,** With echocontrast the apical thrombi are delineated and appear as dark (shadowed) masses. Echocontrast is commonly used to differentiate thrombus from intracardiac tumor. In an intracardiac tumor, presence of contrast within the mass denotes perfusion of the tumor.

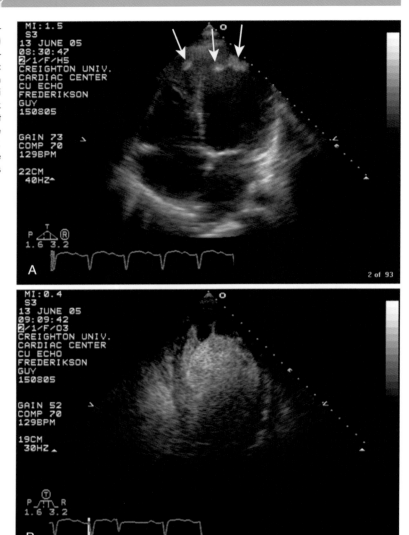

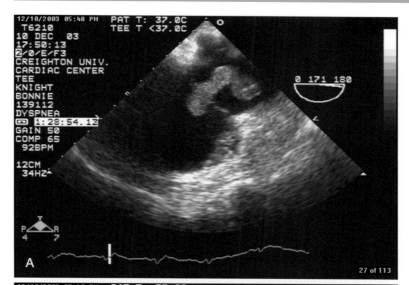

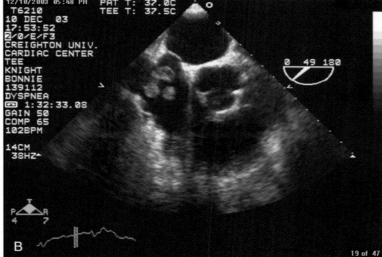

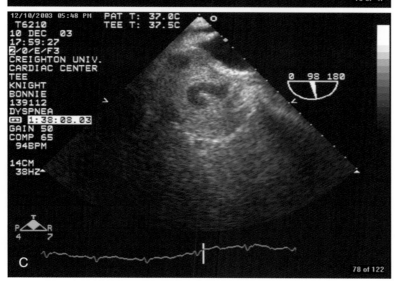

FIGURE 2-10 A, Lower esophageal long-axis view of the right heart showing a large wormlike mass traversing the tricuspid valve consistent with thrombus in transit. **B,** The extensive mobile thrombus is demonstrated again in a midesophageal short-axis view. **C,** Bicaval transesophageal view during saline contrast injection demonstrating again the mobile thrombus (appears shaded) within the right atrium. This patient was undergoing preoperative evaluation before hip surgery and had been relatively immobile for several weeks. She complained of progressive dyspnea on exertion and right leg swelling for the 2 weeks prior to her examination. She received I.V. TPA and a heparin infusion. On follow-up echocardiography approximately 24 hours later, the thrombus was no longer present. The patient had a complete recovery.

FIGURE 2-11 Transthoracic parasternal long- (**A**) and short-axis (**B**) views showing a mass (*asterisks*) within the RV, adherent to the myocardium, extending from the apex to the RVOT. This patient had metastatic renal cell carcinoma. **C,** The tumor is demonstrated again within the RV in this transverse transesophageal view. This patient received chemotherapy, and the tumor metastases were no longer evident on echocardiography after completion of his treatment.

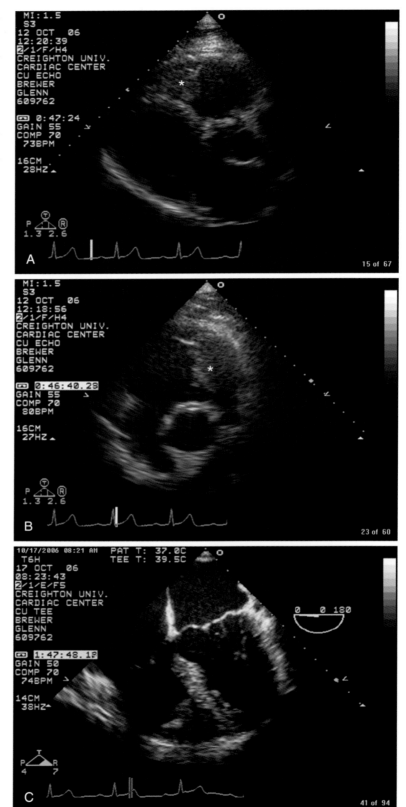

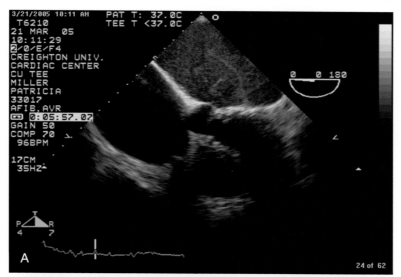

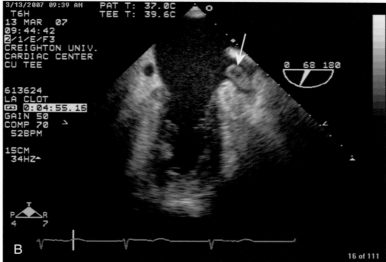

FIGURE 2-12 A, Transverse transesophageal image in a patient with atrial fibrillation. The atria are markedly enlarged and there is significant spontaneous echo contrast visualized within the left atrium. **B,** Transesophageal longitudinal, two-chamber view revealing a large thrombus (*arrow*) within the left atrial appendage in another patient with atrial fibrillation.

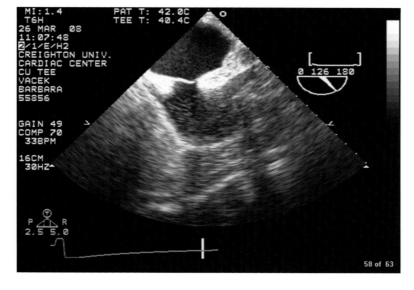

FIGURE 2-13 Longitudinal transesophageal view demonstrating a dumbbell-shaped atrial septum consistent with lipomatous hypertrophy of the septum. Note that fatty infiltration has spared the fossa ovalis.

FIGURE 2-14 A, Left atrial myxoma, the most common intracardiac tumor, is seen in this transthoracic four-chamber view attached to the interatrial septum by a short stalk. This is the most frequent location and attachment site of a cardiac myxoma. **B,** Transesophageal long-axis view of the same patient that also shows the well-circumscribed myxoma within the left atrium.

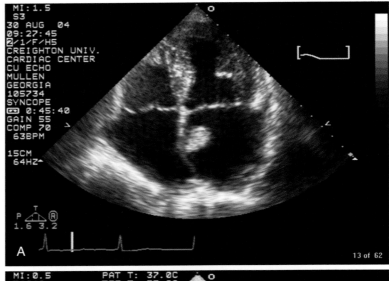

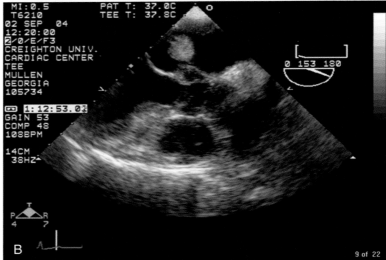

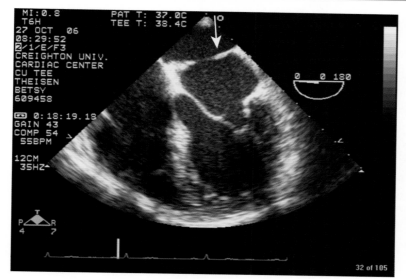

FIGURE 2-15 Transverse transesophageal image of cor triatriatum. The linear echodensity (*arrow*) traversing the left atrium is a membrane separating the left atrium into two compartments. The anterior cavity connects to the mitral valve, and the pulmonary veins drain into the posterior cavity. Blood flows between the two compartments through fenestrations or through an opening in the membrane. The opening may be small and flow-limiting or large and nonlimiting. In this case, there is no obstruction of flow between the two cavities.

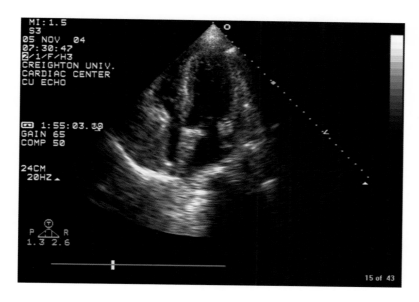

FIGURE 2-16 Two-dimensional echocardiogram of a patient with a large thrombus within the pericardial space seen external to the right atrium and RV. The thrombus is compressing the right atrium, giving it a slitlike appearance. The thrombus was surgically evacuated.

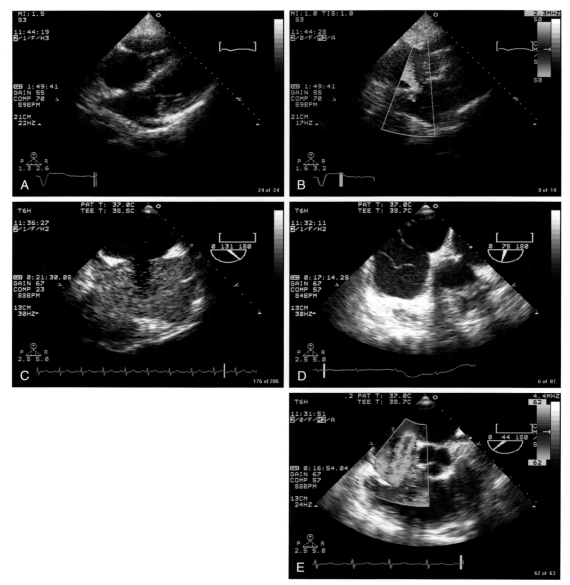

FIGURE 2-17 A, Transthoracic four-chamber subcostal view demonstrating an ostium secundum ASD with biatrial enlargement. **B,** Color flow imaging shows left to right shunting through the ASD. **C,** Transesophageal bicaval view in another patient with an ostium secundum ASD. This image was obtained during a saline contrast study and demonstrates a negative jet secondary to left to right flow across the defect. **D,** Transesophageal image of a prominent Chiari network within the right atrium of a patient with an ostium secundum ASD. **E,** Midesophageal 45-degree short-axis view in the same patient demonstrating left to right shunting through the ASD with color flow imaging.

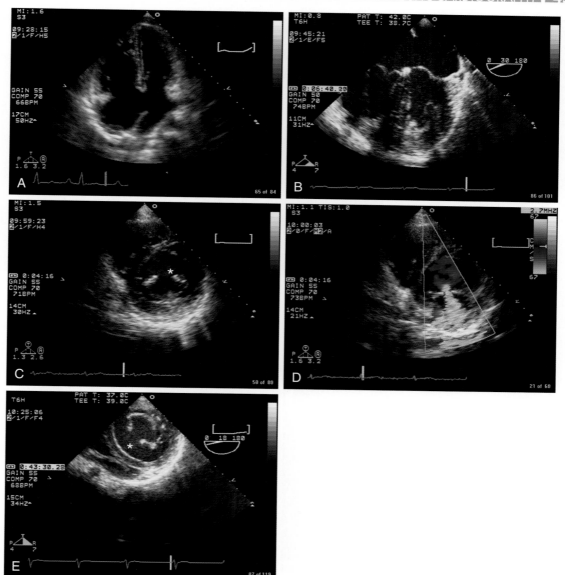

FIGURE 2-18 An ostium primum ASD is shown in this transthoracic apical (**A**) and transesophageal four-chamber (**B**) view. Note apical displacement of the mitral valve, which results in the AV valves lying in the same plane. In this patient the RV is severely enlarged. **C,** An ostium primum ASD is often associated with a cleft mitral valve. This parasternal short-axis view shows a cleft anterior mitral valve leaflet (*asterisk*). **D,** Color flow imaging demonstrates severe mitral regurgitation in this patient. **E,** Transesophageal transgastric short-axis view in the same patient, again demonstrating the cleft in the anterior mitral valve leaflet (*asterisk*).

FIGURE 2-19 A sinus venosus ASD demonstrated on a transesophageal bicaval view. This defect most commonly occurs in the superior aspect of the atrial septum where the SVC enters the right atrium. This defect is commonly associated with anomalous pulmonary venous connections, most often the right upper pulmonary veins draining into the right atrium or SVC.

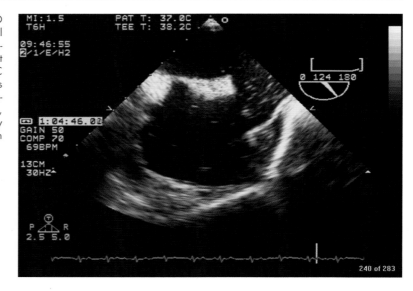

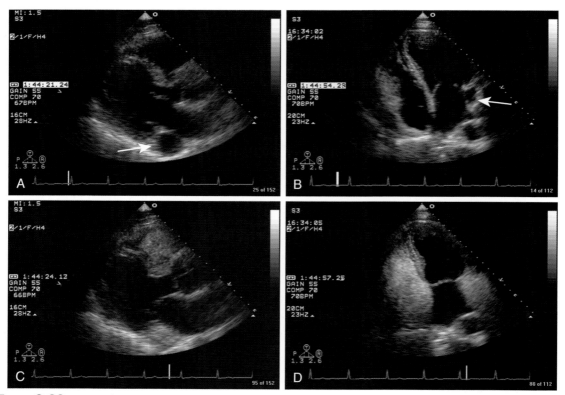

FIGURE 2-20 A, Transthoracic parasternal long-axis view in a patient with a persistent left SVC. Note the dilated coronary sinus (*arrow*) that lies in the left AV groove. The left persistent SVC most commonly drains into the coronary sinus, which results in its enlargement. **B,** Apical four-chamber view in the same patient demonstrating the enlarged coronary sinus (*arrow*). Contrast injection into a peripheral vein in the left arm results in opacification of the coronary sinus and then the right atrium and ventricle, which confirms the presence of a persistent left SVC. Parasternal long-axis (**C**) and apical four-chamber (**D**) views after contrast injection.

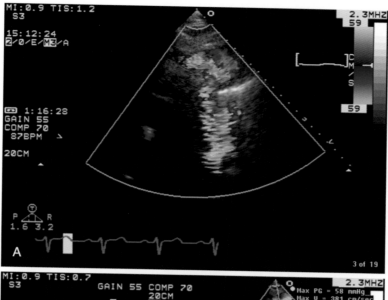

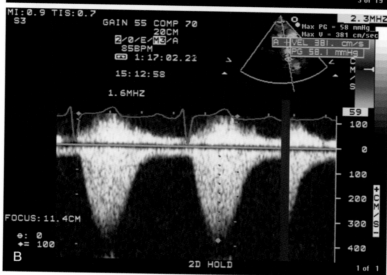

FIGURE 2-21 A, Transthoracic suprasternal notch view demonstrating turbulent flow through an aortic coarctation using color flow imaging. **B,** Continuous wave Doppler demonstrates a gradient of 58 mm Hg across the coarctation. Coarctation of the aorta is commonly associated with a bicuspid aortic valve.

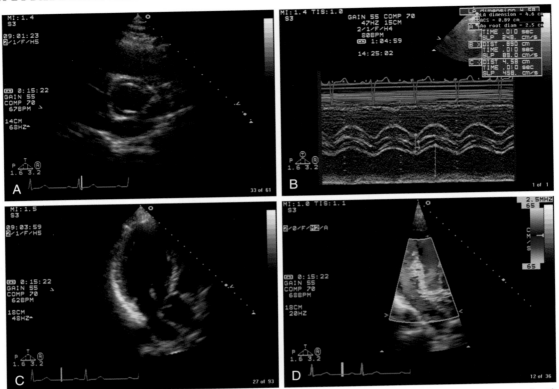

FIGURE 2-22 A, A bicuspid aortic valve during systole in a parasternal short-axis view. This has the appearance of a "fish mouth." **B,** M-mode image of a bicuspid aortic valve. Note the eccentric closure line of the aortic valve. **C,** and **D,** Apical three-chamber view in a patient with a bicuspid aortic valve and severe eccentric aortic regurgitation. Note the eccentric closure line with prolapse of the anterior leaflet. This has resulted in severe posteriorly directed aortic regurgitation.

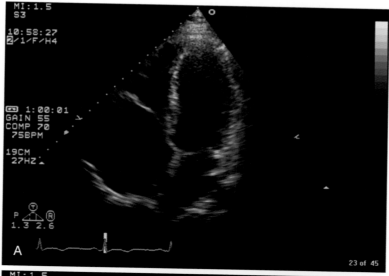

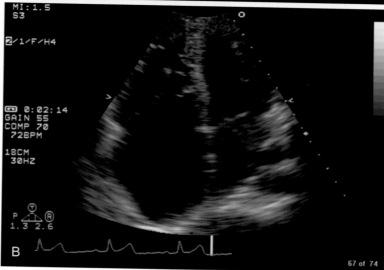

FIGURE 2-23 A and **B,** These transthoracic apical four-chamber images demonstrate Ebstein anomaly. In Ebstein anomaly, the septal leaflet of the tricuspid valve inserts more apically within the RV than usual. This results in atrialization of a portion of the RV; thus, the functioning RV is much smaller. This malformation often results in significant tricuspid regurgitation and enlargement of the right-sided chambers compared to the left-sided chambers.

FIGURE 2-24 A, Transthoracic parasternal short-axis view of the aortic valve, RVOT, pulmonic valve, and PA in an adult patient with an isolated PDA. Color flow imaging below the pulmonic valve (*arrow*) within the pulmonary artery demonstrates a persistent connection between the descending thoracic aorta and PA. **B,** Transesophageal imaging of the descending thoracic aorta and left PA in the same patient. Color flow imaging demonstrates left to right shunting through the PDA.

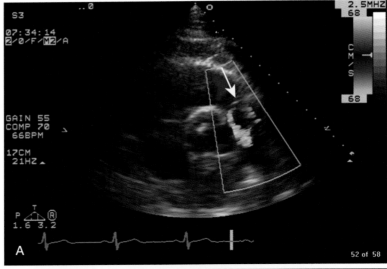

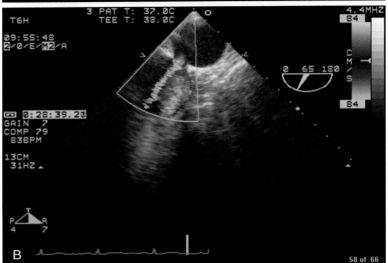

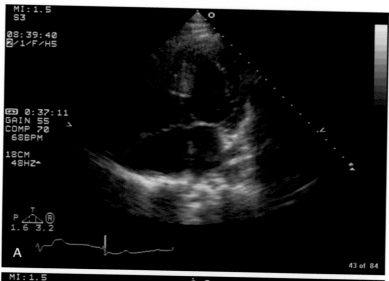

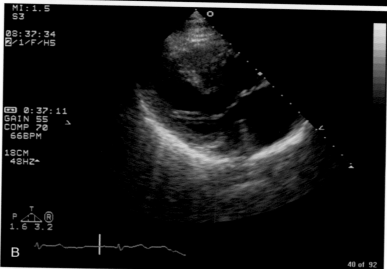

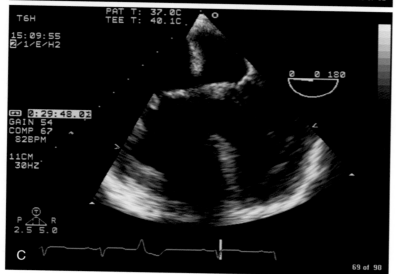

FIGURE 2-25 These images were obtained in an adult Down syndrome patient with an unrepaired complete atrioventricular septal defect. **A,** Transthoracic four-chamber apical view displaying an ostium primum ASD and an inflow VSD. **B,** Parasternal long-axis view showing the inflow VSD between the right and left ventricles. **C,** Transesophageal midesophagus four-chamber view more clearly demonstrating the complete AV septal defect and four-chamber enlargement. Note that there is a common AV valve.

FIGURE 2-26 A, Membranous VSD just below the aortic valve (which is not well seen) visualized in the parasternal long-axis view. Often, the septal leaflet of the tricuspid valve adheres to the ventricular wall, closing or semiclosing the defect. **B,** Apical four-chamber view in another patient with color flow imaging demonstrating left to right shunting through a restrictive membranous VSD.

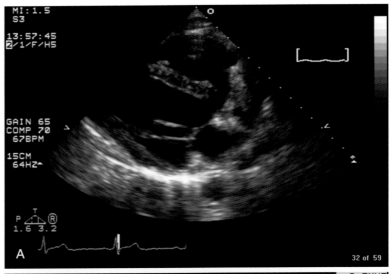

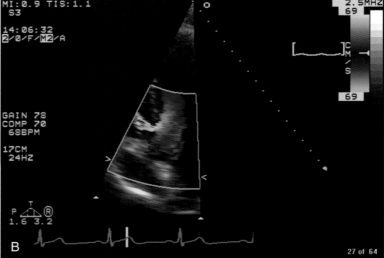

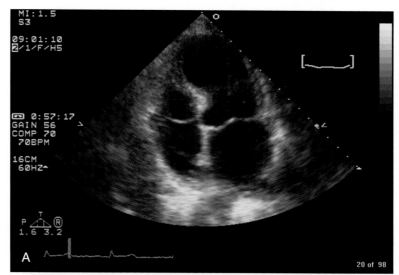

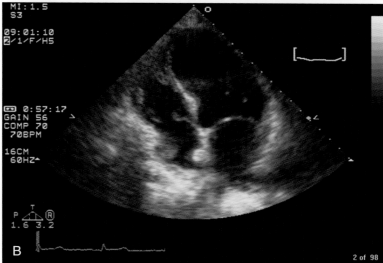

Figure 2-27 Apical transthoracic four-chamber images during systole (**A**) and diastole (**B**) demonstrating akinesis of the entire apex. Biatrial enlargement, left greater than right, is also present. Note that there is very little change in size of the apex between systole and diastole. Additionally, the apical walls do not thicken in systole. Thickening of the proximal septum in systole is apparent.

FIGURE 2-28 These images were obtained in a middle-aged male presenting to the emergency department with near-syncope and generalized malaise. He described severe chest discomfort occurring 4 days earlier. **A,** Apical long-axis view showing a defect (*arrow*) in the midinferolateral wall. **B,** Similar view obtained after definity contrast injection that demonstrates extravasation of contrast through the muscular defect. This patient proceeded to emergent surgery and had repair of his free wall rupture, which occurred several days after a completed infarct in that region.

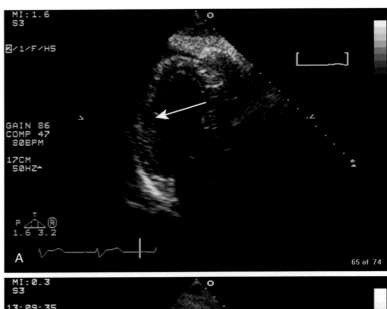

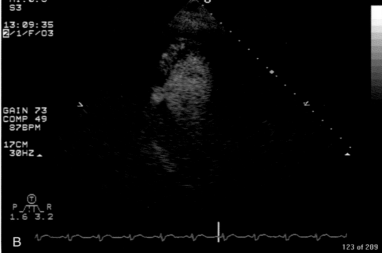

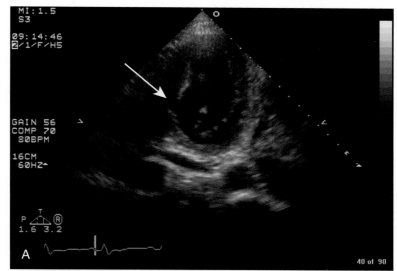

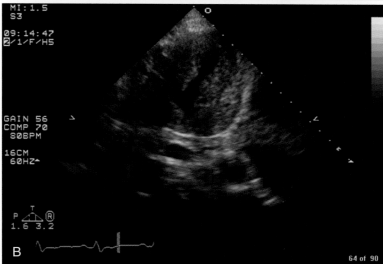

FIGURE 2-29 An 80-year-old female developed pulmonary edema and CHF after being managed medically for a non-STEMI. A transthoracic echocardiogram was obtained. These apical four-chamber images taken during diastole (**A**) and systole (**B**) show a muscular ventricular septal rupture (*arrow*). Note there is also marked LVH.

FIGURE 2-30 A, Apical long-axis transthoracic image obtained in a 50-year-old male with a completed inferior infarct. Rupture of the posteromedial papillary muscle is shown (*arrow*). **B,** This apical four-chamber image demonstrates the ruptured papillary muscle attached via the chordae tendineae to the mitral valve leaflets. The patient underwent emergent surgery and mitral valve replacement. **C,** This echocardiogram was obtained 1 year later in the same patient. He developed an aneurysm of the midinferior wall, shown here in an apical two-chamber view.

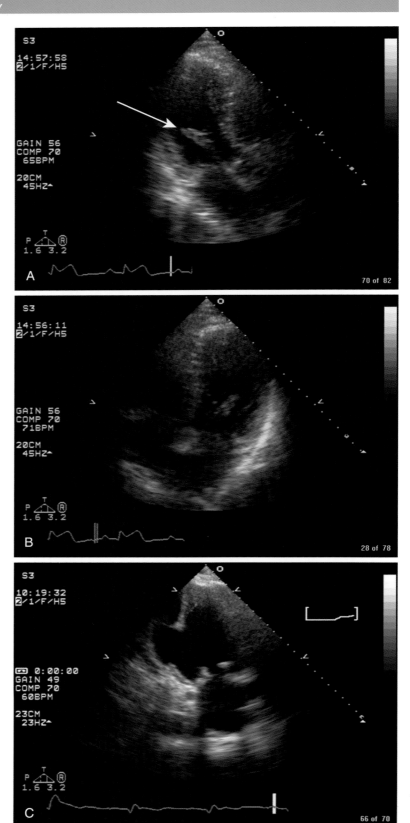

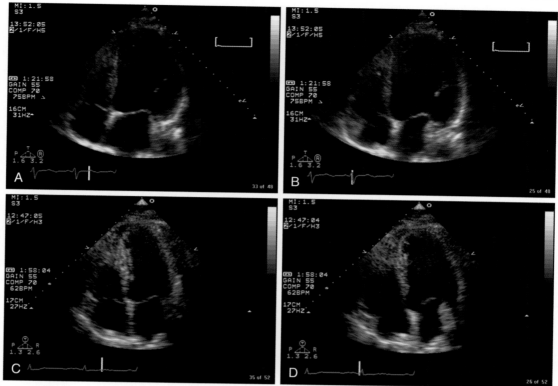

FIGURE 2-31 Echocardiographic findings in a 40-year-old male presenting with chronic angina and progressive dyspnea on exertion. Systolic (**A**) and diastolic (**B**) apical four-chamber images showing marked spherical left ventricular dilation and global hypokinesia. Ejection fraction was estimated at 20% to 25%. The patient had a chronically totally occluded LMCA diagnosed at cardiac catheterization. Systolic (**C**) and diastolic (**D**) images 9 months after the patient underwent CABG surgery; note the left ventricular cavity has strikingly decreased in size and the left ventricular function has markedly improved. Ejection fraction was estimated at 40% to 45%.

FIGURE 2-32 A, A large ostium secundum ASD is easily visualized in this bicaval view obtained during a TEE. Color flow imaging displays left to right shunting through the defect. **B,** An esophageal basal short-axis view of the aortic valve, RVOT, pulmonic valve, and PA (*arrow*) in the same patient. Note the marked enlargement of the RVOT and PA secondary to volume overload from the ASD.

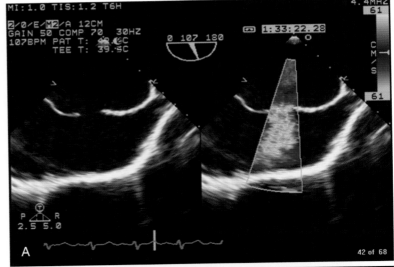

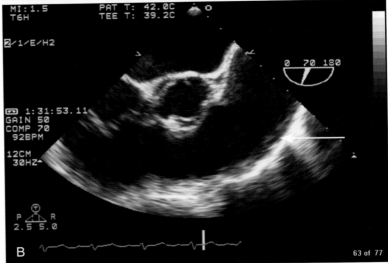

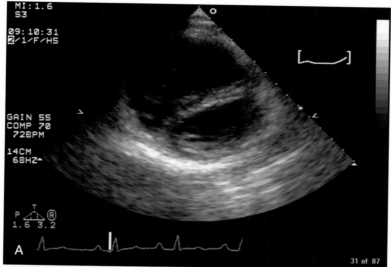

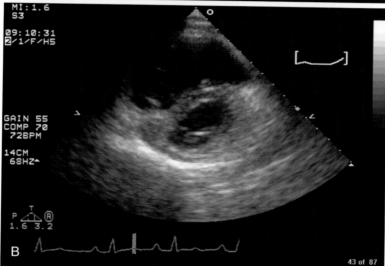

FIGURE 2-33 Diastolic (**A**) and systolic (**B**) 2D parasternal short-axis images in a patient with severe pulmonary hypertension. Note the massive enlargement of the RV, the flattened interventricular septum in systole and diastole, and the resulting D-shaped LV. In isolated right ventricular volume overload, the interventricular septum is flattened during diastole but not during systole.

FIGURE 2-34 A, Transesophageal two-chamber view demonstrating a flail segment of the posterior mitral valve leaflet. **B,** Transesophageal long-axis view of the LV again demonstrating the flail posterior mitral valve leaflet. This resulted in severe eccentric mitral regurgitation directed toward the interatrial septum. This patient underwent successful repair of the mitral valve.

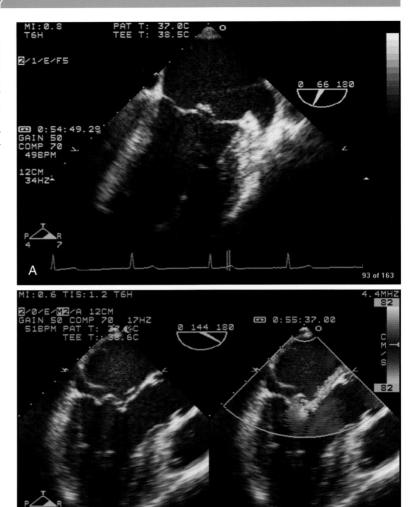

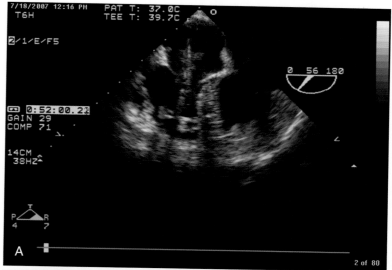

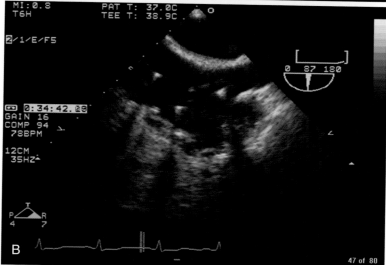

FIGURE 2-35 TEE in a middle-aged female with persistently positive blood cultures growing *Staphylococcus aureus*. **A,** Midgastric transesophageal view demonstrating an ICD lead traversing the tricuspid valve. Note the shaggy thickened appearance of the entire lead with multiple large mobile echodensities attached to the portion of the lead within the RV apex consistent with endocarditis. **B,** Bicaval transesophageal view in the same patient showing the ICD lead entering the right atrium from the SVC. Multiple mobile vegetations are also noted attached to the ICD wire within the right atrium, which were not well visualized on transthoracic imaging. The patient underwent device explantation and lead extraction combined with I.V. antibiotics, which was curative.

FIGURE 2-36 Echocardiographic images demonstrating bileaflet mitral valve endocarditis. **A,** Apical four-chamber view showing irregular nodular thickening of the mitral valve leaflets. **B,** Parasternal long-axis view of the LV in the same patient. Note the large relatively sessile vegetation attached to atrial surface of the posterior mitral valve leaflet. The vegetation of the anterior mitral valve leaflet is not as well visualized in this view. **C,** Severe mitral regurgitation was present in this patient.

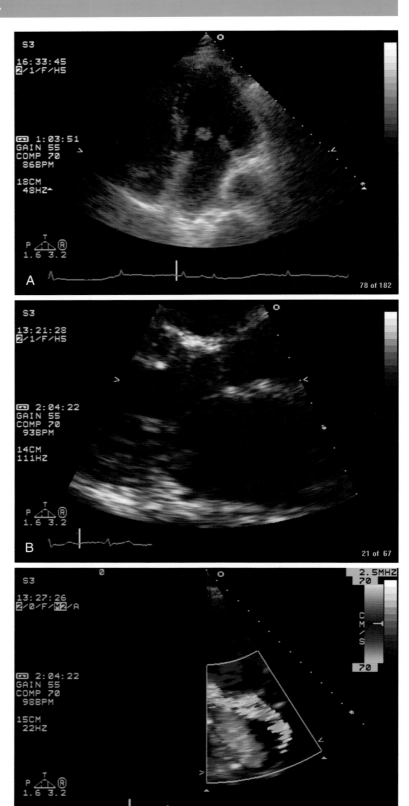

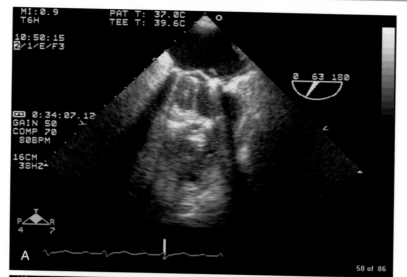

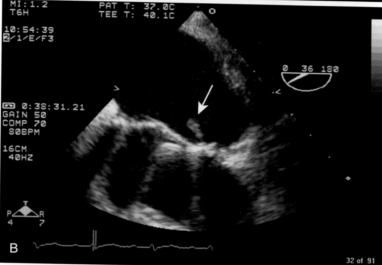

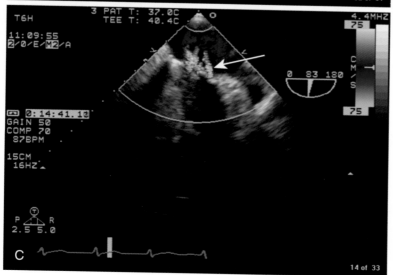

FIGURE 2-37 Transesophageal images in a patient with endocarditis of his St. Jude mitral valve prosthesis. **A,** This still frame was captured at the onset of systole. Note the prosthetic leaflets are closed. Attached to the atrial side of the prosthetic valve sewing ring is a large mobile echodensity consistent with vegetation. **B,** A close-up view of the vegetation (*arrow*) attached to the edge of the prosthesis. **C,** Color flow imaging demonstrating the expected three jets of minimal regurgitation that occur with closure of the leaflets. Also note the presence of mitral regurgitation occurring at the site of the vegetation, consistent with a paravalvular leak (*long arrow*).

FIGURE 2-38 A, Transthoracic parasternal long-axis image in a patient with rheumatic mitral stenosis. The mitral leaflets are thickened with minimal calcification. Here, in diastole, the leaflets dome into the LV. The anterior leaflet has the classic form of a hockey stick. **B,** Apical four-chamber image in the same patient showing the generalized thickening of the mitral valve leaflets and their restricted opening in diastole. The left atrium is severely enlarged.

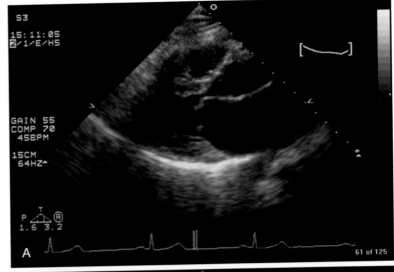

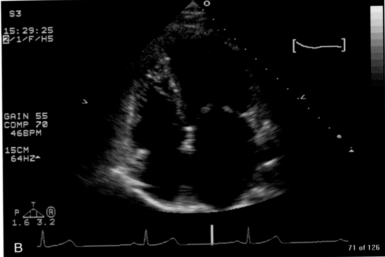

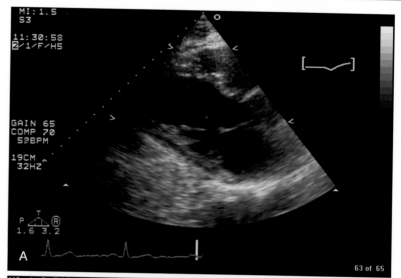

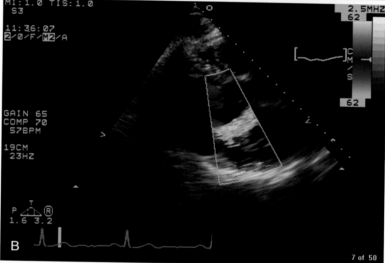

FIGURE 2-39 Ruptured chordae tendineae. **A,** Parasternal long-axis view displaying ruptured chordae tendineae attached to the posterior mitral valve leaflet, which resulted in a flail segment of the posterior leaflet. This patient presented with progressive shortness of breath over several days with pulmonary edema. **B,** Severe mitral regurgitation was evident by color flow Doppler imaging.

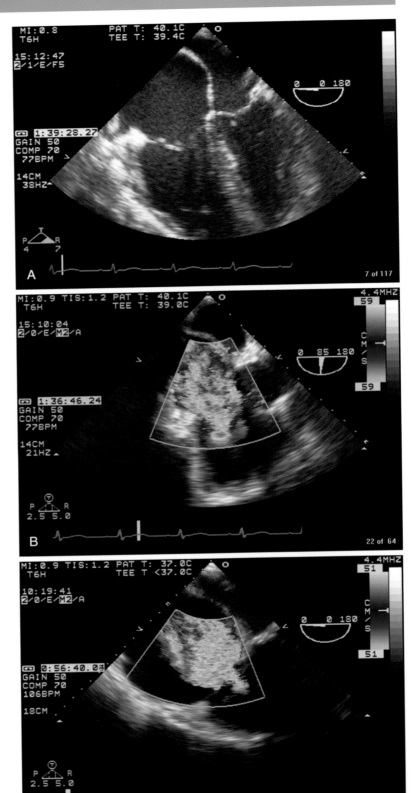

FIGURE 2-40 A, Transesophageal four-chamber still frame in a patient with severe tricuspid regurgitation. The RV and right atrium are dilated. The atrial septum bows to the left, consistent with high right atrial pressure. **B,** Color flow imaging in the same patient showing severe tricuspid regurgitation filling the right atrium. **C,** A transesophageal still frame image in another patient with severe central tricuspid regurgitation. The tricuspid annulus is dilated and the right atrium is massively enlarged.

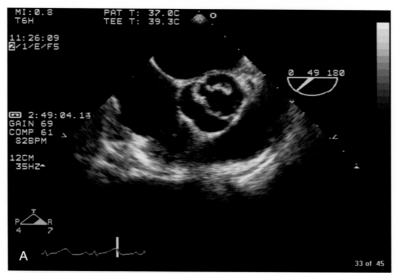

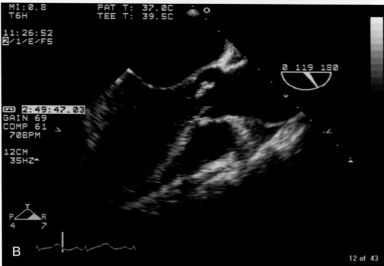

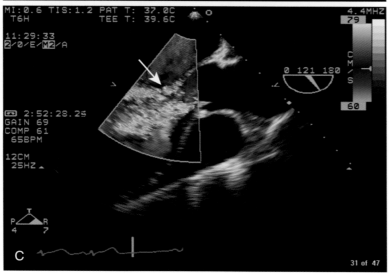

FIGURE 2-41 Endocarditis of a bicuspid aortic valve. **A,** Transesophageal short-axis view of a bicuspid aortic valve showing thickening and increased echogenicity of the leaflets suspicious for endocarditis. **B,** Transesophageal long-axis view in the same patient. A mobile vegetation is evident on the anterior cusp of the bicuspid aortic valve. **C,** Perforation of the anterior cusp of the valve demonstrated with color flow imaging. Note the two jets of aortic regurgitation, one through the perforation (*arrow*) and the other through the valve orifice.

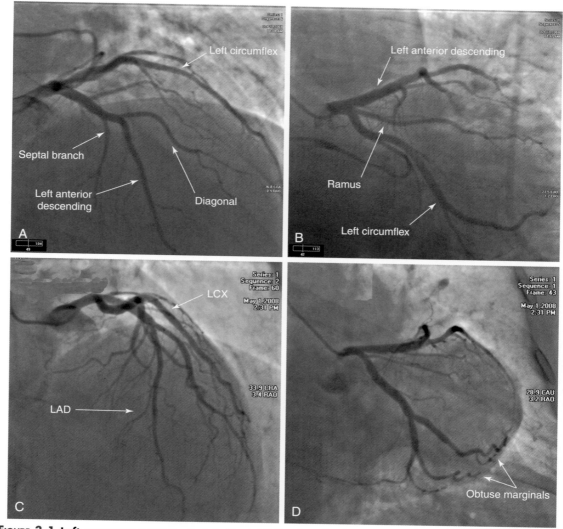

FIGURE 3-1 Left coronary system. A, A Judkins left 3.5 catheter has been advanced to the LMCA ostium via the right radial approach. This projection is obtained in the AP cranial view. The LMCA arises in the normal location from the left sinus of Valsalva. The LAD travels down toward the bottom of the image. The major branches that arise from this artery are the septal penetrators and the diagonals. The LCX is located across the top of the image and moves toward the right. This view has significant overlap of the circumflex branches, noted by the double density of contrast media. **B,** The AP caudal projection demonstrates the bifurcation of the LAD and LCX systems and is used to look for ostial stenoses. The LCX gives rise to major branches that are termed *obtuse marginals*. In this image, a branch occurs between the LAD and LCX, arising from the LMCA. When present, the artery is named the ramus intermediate. **C,** An AP cranial view of another normal LAD. This image allows better visualization of the mid- and distal LAD. In this patient, the first diagonal is nearly the same size as the LAD. **D,** Finally, another AP caudal projection demonstrating the bifurcation of the LAD and LCX systems. There is no significant CAD present in this patient. The LCX system is seen as it travels toward the bottom right corner of this image. The LAD is located at the top of the image moving horizontally across.

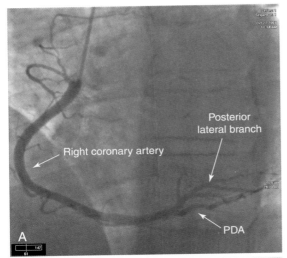

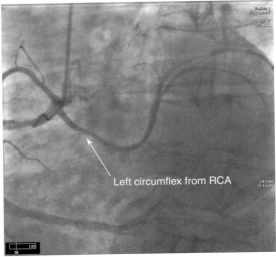

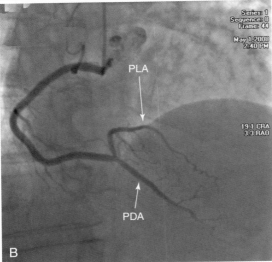

FIGURE 3-2 Right coronary system. A, A Judkins right 4.0 catheter is placed at the ostium of the RCA, and an angiogram is obtained in the straight LAO projection. No significant disease is noted. This is a right dominant coronary system; the PDA arises from the distal RCA. **B,** This is an AP cranial view of another RCA. The bifurcation of the posterior descending coronary artery and posterolateral coronary artery is best visualized in this view.

FIGURE 3-3 Anomalous LCX. Diagnostic cardiac catheterization in a patient with unstable angina. The LCX arises off the right coronary cusp from the same orifice as the RCA (anomalous origin of the LCX).

The most common coronary anomaly is separate ostia of the LCX and LAD arising from the left sinus of Valsalva. This is followed by the LCX arising from the RCA or right sinus of Valsalva.

Most coronary anomalies are clinically silent; however, if the LMCA arises from the pulmonary trunk or aberrantly courses between the great vessels, an increased association with sudden death, myocardial ischemia, and endocarditis is seen.

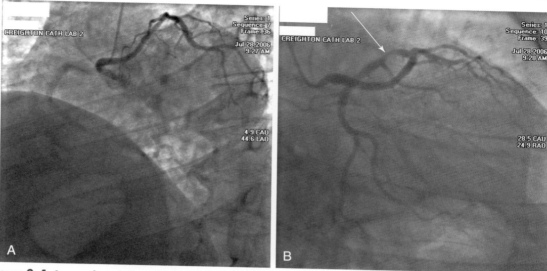

FIGURE 3-4 Anomalous left main from the right coronary cusp. A, This image is obtained in the LAO projection. A Judkins right catheter has been advanced into the aorta from the right radial artery. As contrast medium is injected, there is faint filling of the RCA coming toward the left side of the image. The catheter, however, is in the ostium of the LMCA. The LMCA is anomalous and transverses across the heart muscle and bifurcates into the LAD and LCX. In this view, it appears that the artery courses anterior to the aorta, but further imaging should be performed to confirm this positioning. **B,** This image is obtained in the RAO projection. This clearly demonstrates that the LMCA is very long and extends to the left ventricular side before it bifurcates. There is severe stenosis of the proximal LCX (*arrow*).

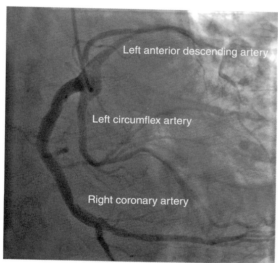

FIGURE 3-5 Single coronary artery. A Judkins right 4.0 coronary catheter is noted in the right coronary cusp on this LAO projection. As the contrast enters the artery, all three of the major coronary arteries are visualized arising from the same common trunk. The RCA follows the standard course toward the inferior border of the heart. The LCX is located in the middle of the image and travels to the lateral wall of the ventricle. The LAD is toward the back of the image and is recognized secondary to the presence of septal branches. This anomaly is rare, occurring in 0.02% of the population.

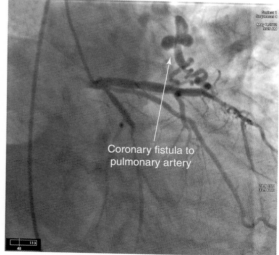

FIGURE 3-6 Coronary artery fistula. LAO view of the left coronary system during diagnostic catheterization. Note the fistula from the LAD to the PA. This is the most common type of coronary artery fistula. Other connections include from a coronary artery to the right ventricle, right atrium, or coronary sinus.

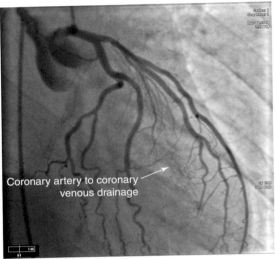

FIGURE 3-7 Coronary artery to coronary venous drainage. A Judkins left 4.0 catheter has been placed in the ostium of the LMCA via the femoral approach. The angiogram is obtained in the RAO caudal projection. As the contrast medium enters the left coronary circulation, staining is noted in the middle of the cardiac silhouette that partially clears with ventricular systole. This is consistent with coronary artery to coronary venous drainage. The coronary venous drainage occurs through the thebesian system directly into the ventricles.

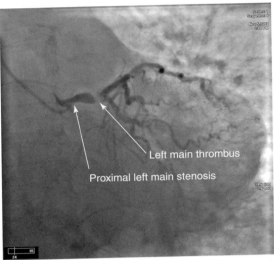

FIGURE 3-8 Left main stenosis with thrombus. A Judkins left 3.5 catheter is placed in the LMCA ostium from the right radial approach. In the AP caudal projection, a lesion is noted at the origin of the LMCA. Comparing the diameter of the vessel proximal to and distal to the lesion, a significant narrowing is noted. The most striking portion of this angiogram is the hazy lucent portion of the artery at the bifurcation of the LAD and LCX, secondary to a large thrombus. In the cine angiograms, the flow into the distal vessels is slightly impaired. An additional thrombus is noted in the mid-LCX. In addition, the RCA is filled late by collaterals, demonstrating that the proximal portion of the artery is likely occluded. The entire coronary circulation is compromised by the thrombus.

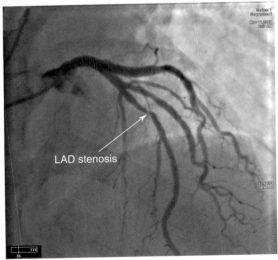

FIGURE 3-9 Left anterior descending artery stenosis. A Judkins left coronary catheter is positioned in the LMCA ostium from the right radial approach. The camera is positioned in the AP cranial projection. In the middle of the frame, a significant flow-limiting stenosis is seen in the mid-LAD. This lesion is located after the bifurcation of the first diagonal branch. Comparing the luminal diameter in the arterial segment proximal to and distal to the lesion, there is an approximate 90% to 99% narrowing of the artery.

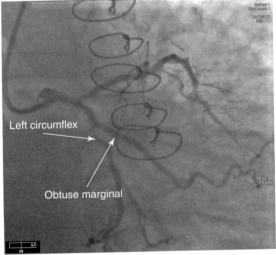

FIGURE 3-10 Left circumflex artery stenosis. This angiogram is obtained via the radial approach in the LAO caudal projection. This view is ideal for separating the ostia of the LAD and LCX. The LAD is the more superior vessel and travels to the left of the image. The LCX is the lower vessel and travels toward the bottom of the image. A 90% to 99% lesion is present in the midportion of the LCX just after the takeoff of the first obtuse marginal branch. The area appears to be slightly more radiolucent than the surrounding vessel. This is an irregular plaque producing significant narrowing.

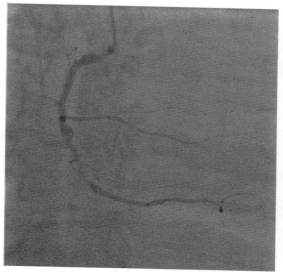

FIGURE 3-11 Right coronary artery stenosis. This angiogram of the RCA is obtained in the straight LAO projection. A severe obstructive lesion is seen in the midsegment of the vessel. The segment of artery distal to the large acute marginal branch is diseased as it enters the area with the severe lesion. The distal vessel is small but relatively free of disease.

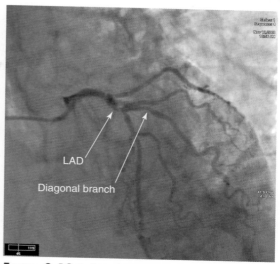

FIGURE 3-12 Left anterior descending/diagonal stenosis. The image has been obtained in the AP cranial projection. In the middle of the frame, a significant stenosis of the LAD involving the bifurcation of a large diagonal branch is seen. This stenosis makes percutaneous intervention more complicated because there is a risk that flow will be compromised within this side branch.

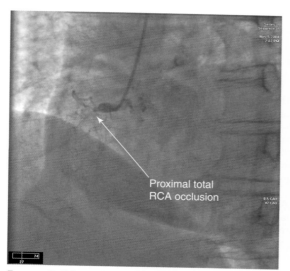

FIGURE 3-13 Total right coronary artery occlusion. A Judkins right 4.0 catheter is positioned at the ostium of the RCA. This image is obtained in the LAO view. The artery is totally occluded proximally. The lesion is said to be in the proximal portion of the vessel because it occurs before the first major acute marginal branch. The mid-RCA is defined as the portion of the artery from the end of the proximal segment to the next major acute marginal branch. The distal RCA is located from the end of the midsegment to the bifurcation of the PDA.

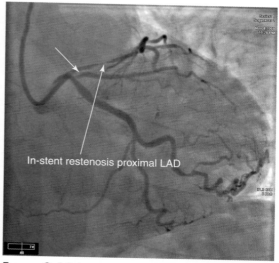

FIGURE 3-14 In-stent restenosis of left anterior descending artery. An XB guiding catheter is present in the LMCA ostium from the radial artery approach. This image was obtained in the AP caudal projection. Before contrast injection, a stent can be visualized in the proximal portion of the LAD. A significant narrowing within the stent is consistent with in-stent restenosis. The LCX is without significant disease. However, there is a significant ostial lesion (*short arrow*) of the first obtuse marginal branch.

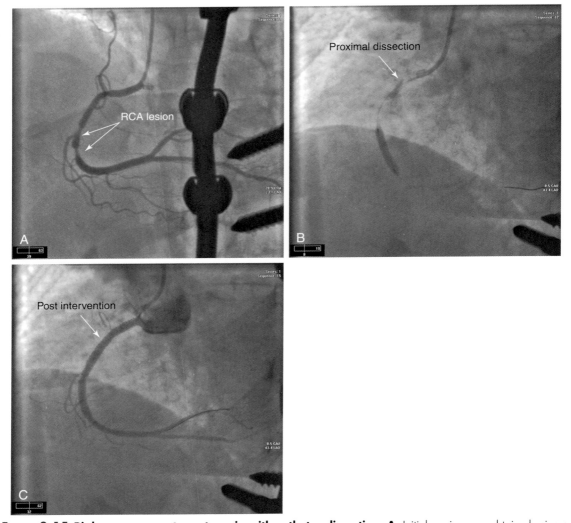

FIGURE 3-15 Right coronary artery stenosis with catheter dissection. A, Initial angiograms obtained using a diagnostic catheter via the right radial approach demonstrate severe lesions in the midportion of the RCA. **B,** In the second angiogram in this series, a Judkins right 4.0 guiding catheter is in the ostium of the RCA. A 0.014-inch wire has been advanced through the lesion and into the distal vessel. A balloon is inflated at the site of the original lesion. Note the contrast persistent within the proximal vessel. A type D coronary dissection is noted. This occurs when the guide wire becomes subintimal and then reenters the lumen more distally. The dissection then propagates in a spiral fashion down the arterial wall. **C,** To prevent further propagation of the dissection and coronary occlusion, the injured site is often covered with a stent, as shown in the final sequence.

Dissections are categorized by NHLBI classification as type A to F. Type A and B dissections can often be managed conservatively, whereas type C through F require additional treatment. Type A dissections demonstrate a small radiolucent area within the coronary lumen during contrast injection but no persistence of contrast in the vessel. Type B dissections show a "parallel" tract or double lumen separated by a radiolucent band during angiography without residual contrast when the injection is completed. A Type C dissection appears with contrast media located outside the coronary lumen. This is termed the *extraluminal cap.* There is contrast media present after the dye has cleared from the main lumen. Type D dissections are spiral dissections often with contrast staining of the false lumen. Type E dissections appear as new persistent filling defects within the coronary lumen. Type F dissections cause total occlusion of the vessel without distal flow.

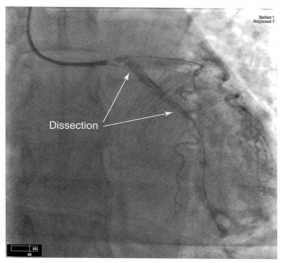

FIGURE 3-16 LMCA and LCX dissection. An XB guiding catheter is visualized at the ostium of the LMCA. A type E dissection of the LCX was caused by the diagnostic coronary catheter; this dissection propagated proximally to the LMCA. Two wires are present: one in the LAD and the other in the LCX. These wires maintained flow into the distal arterial system. The patient was taken to the operating room for emergent CABG surgery.

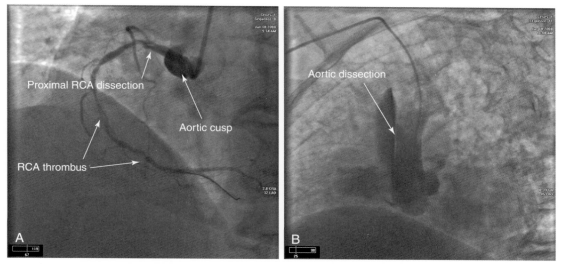

FIGURE 3-17 Aortic cusp/root dissection. A, An Amplatz left guiding catheter is near the ostium of the RCA. A 0.014-inch wire is present in preparation for intervention because significant stenosis and thrombus are present within the vessel. A dissection flap is noted in the proximal artery and likely begins at the ostial-aortic junction. As the angiogram is obtained, contrast enters into the aortic wall and stains the cusp. **B,** The dissection at the cusp has now propagated superiorly and is involving the proximal portion of the aortic root. This often requires immediate surgical repair, as this is a Stanford class A aortic dissection.

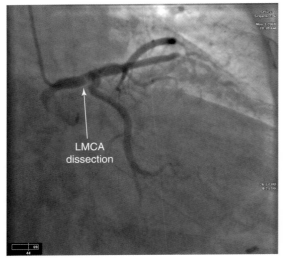

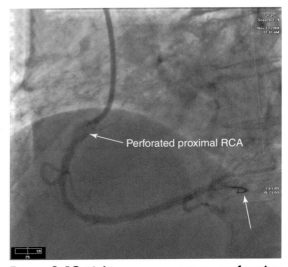

LMCA
dissection

Perforated proximal RCA

FIGURE 3-18 Left main coronary artery dissection. A catheter is positioned in the LMCA via the right radial approach. The angiogram is obtained in the AP caudal view. Note that prior to injection, contrast material is already present in the artery at the tip of the catheter, suggestive of a coronary artery dissection. As the contrast is injected, the contrast material does not clear from the proximal segment. In addition, a radiolucent line is apparent in the distal portion of the LMCA. This is the dissection flap.

FIGURE 3-19 Right coronary artery perforation with rotational atherectomy device. In this angiogram, intervention is being performed on the RCA. A Judkins right guiding catheter is positioned above the ostium of the RCA. A 0.014-inch wire is present and has been advanced into the distal vessel (*arrow*). The diagnostic coronary angiogram demonstrated a significant stenosis in the proximal portion of the artery, which was heavily calcified. Due to the heavy calcification, it was determined that debulking of the lesion before stent implantation would improve the result. Debulking of heavily calcified lesions can be done with rotational atherectomy. With a rotational atherectomy device on the wire, several passes are made through the lesion. Afterwards, a repeat angiogram is obtained. The proximal RCA has been perforated and contrast is noted outside the vessel lumen. This is treated using prolonged balloon inflations in the affected segment until the perforation is sealed. In addition, a covered stent may be placed over the perforated segment.

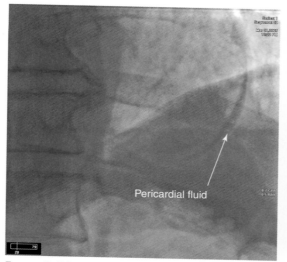

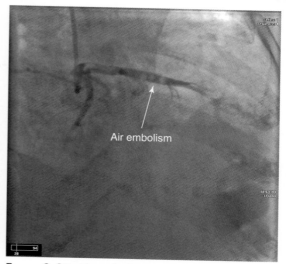

FIGURE 3-20 Coronary perforation with pericardial staining. This is a postintervention angiogram in the straight AP projection. The patient underwent intervention to the LAD and a wire passed outside the vessel lumen. Contrast can be seen in the pericardial space, indicating that the vessel has been perforated.

FIGURE 3-21 Air embolism. A catheter is present in the LMCA via the right radial approach. The image was captured in the RAO caudal projection. The LCX courses down toward the bottom left corner of the image. The LAD travels across the image. The discrete areas of lucency noted in the LAD are air emboli that occurred at the time of contrast injection. The patient is administered high-flow oxygen while the air emboli dissolve.

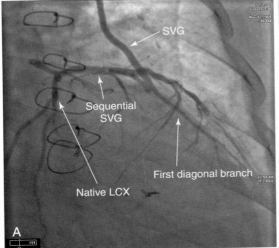

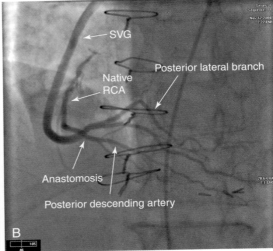

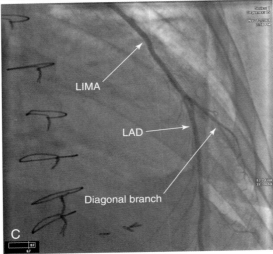

FIGURE 3-22 Coronary artery bypass angiography. A, A Judkins right catheter has been positioned in the ascending aorta from the femoral approach. Notice that this catheter position is higher than would be expected for normal coronary artery origins. Grafts to the left coronary system usually arise from the left side of the aorta, and those to the RCA usually arise from the right side of the aorta. This selective angiogram has been obtained in the RAO caudal view. It demonstrates an SVG that travels from the aorta to the first diagonal branch of the LAD and then in a sequential fashion to the first obtuse marginal branch of the LCX. **B,** The catheter has now been positioned on the right side of the aorta. Again, the position of the catheter is significantly higher than the normal position of the native coronary arteries. This image was obtained in the AP cranial projection. This SVG is to the distal RCA. The native artery fills in a retrograde fashion up to the area of occlusion. The distal vessels of the right coronary circulation, the PDA and PLA, are well visualized and free of significant disease. **C,** The catheter has now been advanced into the left subclavian artery and has been positioned at the ostium of the LIMA. This is the preferred bypass conduit to use for the LAD circulation, because the patency of this graft is 90% at 10 years. The angiogram is obtained in the RAO cranial projection. This allows for adequate visualization of the anastomosis of the mammary artery to the coronary artery. Visualizing the anastomosis is important because many times flow-limiting lesions occur at this site.

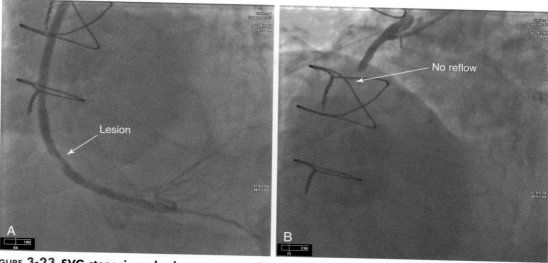

FIGURE 3-23 SVG stenosis and subsequent no reflow. A, An SVG anastomosed to the distal RCA is shown in this LAO cranial view. Note the significant lesion in the distal portion of the graft. Using a distal protection device, the lesion was dilated and a stent was placed. However, after removal of the guidewire, no reflow was noted. **B,** No reflow is likely to occur when a large thrombus burden is present or when intervention has been performed on a degenerated SVG. A lack of reflow is caused by distal embolization into the microcirculation. These vessels are too small to be visualized by angiography; however, because there is no outlet for the contrast material, the dye appears to "hang" in the artery. It is treated by intra-arterial injections of vasodilator medications, such as nicardipine and nitroprusside.

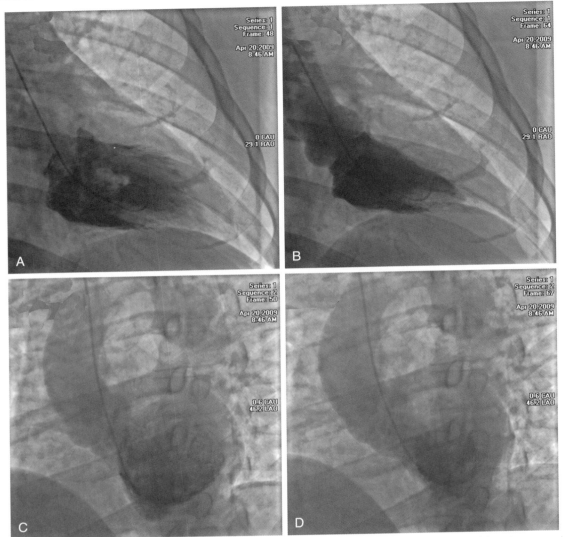

FIGURE 3-24 Left ventriculography. Images obtained in the RAO projection, one in diastole (**A**) and the other in systole (**B**). A pigtail catheter has been placed into the LV through the aortic valve. In diastole, the left ventricular cavity is of normal size and becomes significantly smaller in systole. During systole, all of the myocardial segments contract inward and thicken. There are no regional wall motion abnormalities. Images are also often obtained in the LAO projection, diastole (**C**) and systole (**D**).

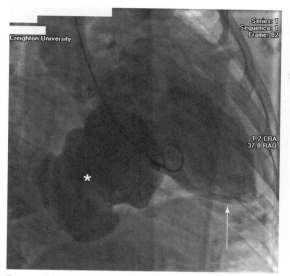

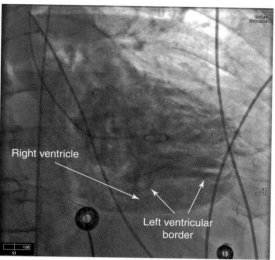

FIGURE 3-25 Giant left ventricular aneurysm. This image is obtained in the RAO projection. A pigtail catheter is in the left ventricular cavity, and contrast medium is injected to visualize the chamber. The apex of the heart is located toward the bottom right edge of the image (*arrow*). The large mass that appears to be arising from the diaphragmatic wall of the LV, is a large left ventricular aneurysm (*asterisk*). The aneurysm has a large opening or neck that distinguishes it from a pseudoaneurysm, which has a narrow neck. This is an unusual location for a left ventricular aneurysm. Common locations for these defects are at the apex and in the anterior wall.

FIGURE 3-26 Post-infarct VSD. Left ventriculogram in an RAO view demonstrating a VSD, which occurred several days after an anteroseptal MI.

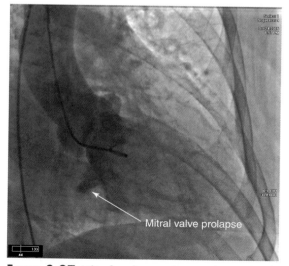

FIGURE 3-27 Mitral valve prolapse. A pigtail catheter has been placed into the LV via the femoral approach. The ventriculogram has been obtained in the RAO projection. The posterior leaflet of the mitral valve is prolapsing into the left atrium. Mild mitral regurgitation is noted.

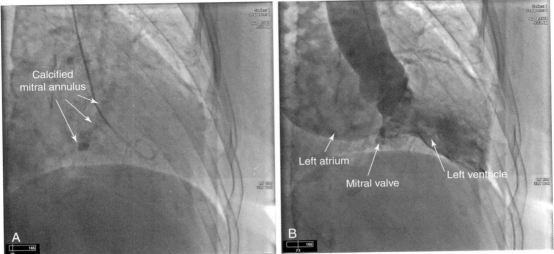

FIGURE 3-28 Mitral annular calcification and mitral regurgitation. A, A pigtail catheter has been placed into the LV via the right radial approach. The large area of calcification in the center of the image represents the annulus of the mitral valve. **B,** As contrast is injected into the ventricle, a significant amount of dye is passing back through the mitral valve into the left atrium indicating moderate to severe mitral regurgitation. The left atrium is severely enlarged. Assessment of mitral regurgitation using contrast angiography is determined in the following manner: Mild (1+): Faint left atrial opacification that clears with each beat and does not opacify the entire left atrium. Moderate (2+): The left atrium is completely opacified after several beats. The left atrium is more opacified than the LV. Moderate to severe (3+): The left atrium is completely opacified and is equal to the left ventricular opacification. Severe (4+): The left atrium is completely opacified after one beat. The left atrium is opacified more than the left ventricle. Opacification of the pulmonary veins is also present.

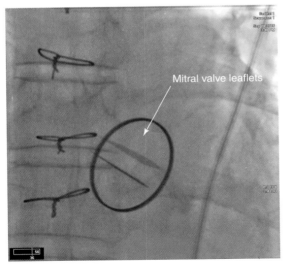

FIGURE 3-29 Prosthetic mitral valve. An AP projection of a normal functioning bileaflet prosthetic mitral valve. On the moving cine loops both leaflets open and close appropriately. The optimal view to determine proper function is the RAO projection.

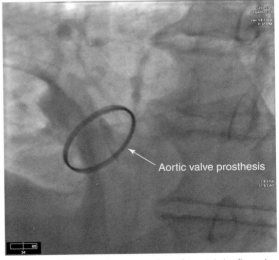

FIGURE 3-30 Prosthetic aortic valve. A bileaflet valve is noted in the aortic position in this radiograph obtained in the LAO projection. In the still frame, the leaflets are captured in the open position. Note that this valve is smaller than the valve that was previously visualized in the mitral position.

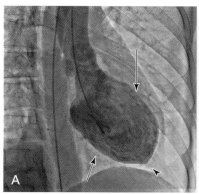 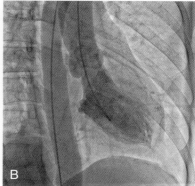

FIGURE 3-31 Dialated cardiomyopathy. Diastole (**A**) and systole (**B**). A pigtail catheter is placed in the left ventricle. This catheter is not in the ideal position because it is located near the mitral valve apparatus. This image, obtained in the RAO projection, allows visualization of the anterolateral (*long arrow*), apical (*arrowhead*), and diaphragmatic (*short arrow*) segments of myocardium. As contrast medium is injected into the ventricle, the movement of the myocardial segments is determined by the reduction of the ventricular cavity size, allowing estimation of left ventricular systolic function. Each individual segment is also evaluated for contractility and described accordingly. *Hypokinesis* is defined as reduced inward motion during systole. *Akinesis* is the absence of inward motion during systole. *Dyskinesis* is defined as paradoxical outward motion during systole. The LV in this image is dilated; overall contractility is moderately impaired. The ejection fraction is estimated at approximately 30%.

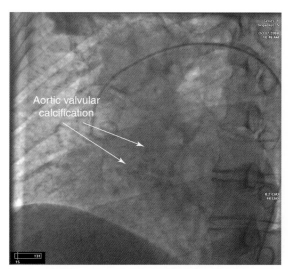

FIGURE 3-32 Aortic valve calcification with severe aortic insufficiency. A pigtail catheter has been advanced into the ascending aorta from the femoral approach. Before injection of contrast medium, a radiolucent area is noted at the location of the aortic valve, representing heavy calcification of the aortic valve apparatus. As contrast is injected, the LV quickly becomes filled at the same density of the aorta, demonstrating severe aortic insufficiency. In addition, the aortic root is mildly dilated.

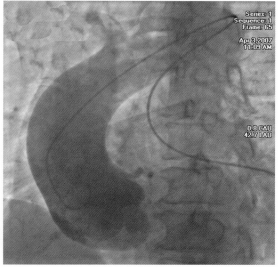

FIGURE 3-33 Dilated aortic root. In this image, a pigtail catheter has been advanced into the ascending aorta via the femoral approach. The course of the catheter appears unusual as it comes up to and crosses the aortic arch secondary to severe tortuosity of the aorta. After contrast injection, the aortic root and ascending aorta are noted to be quite enlarged. Compare the size of aortic root to the size of the aortic arch after the innominate artery.

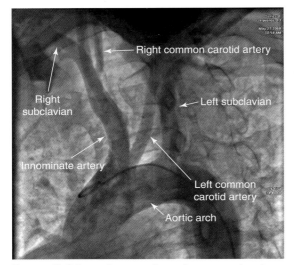

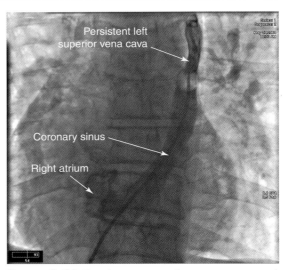

FIGURE 3-34 Bovine aortic arch. A pigtail catheter has been advanced into the ascending aorta via the femoral approach, and this image has been obtained in the AP projection. The normal orientation of the great vessels includes three separate ostia: the right innominate, then the left common carotid, and finally the left subclavian arteries. In this patient, the origin of the right innominate artery is located in the proper location; however, the origin of the left carotid artery is from a shared common trunk with the right innominate artery, termed a *bovine arch*. This orientation occurs in 15% of patients. A less common finding is to have the left common carotid artery originate from the innominate artery proper, which occurs in approximately 10% of patients.

FIGURE 3-35 Persistent superior vena cava. A balloon-tipped catheter has been advanced through the cardiac silhouette. The catheter has passed through the IVC into the right atrium through the coronary sinus into a persistent left SVC. Persistent left SVC is the most common abnormality of the thoracic venous system, present in 0.3% of the population. It is often associated with other cardiac abnormalities, such as VSD and ASD.

FIGURE 3-36 Fibromuscular dysplasia. Image of the abdominal aorta obtained in the AP projection. A pigtail catheter has been advanced from the radial artery to the level of the renal arteries. The right renal artery appears to have a "string-of-beads" appearance (*arrow*), which suggests fibromuscular dysplasia (not optimally imaged here). This autosomal dominant disorder, usually discovered between the ages of 14 and 50 years, is characterized by fibrous thickening of any of the layers of the arterial wall. Most commonly the medial layer is affected and causes narrowing of the arterial lumen. If intervention is needed in these cases, angioplasty is most often done without the need for stenting.

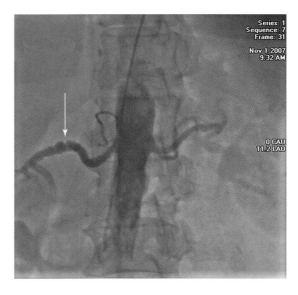

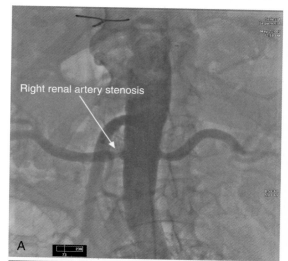

Right renal artery stenosis

A

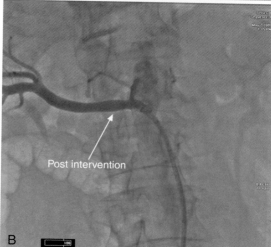

Post intervention

B

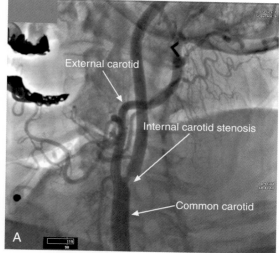

External carotid

Internal carotid stenosis

Common carotid

A

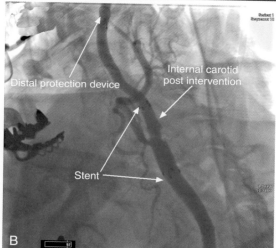

Distal protection device

Internal carotid post intervention

Stent

B

FIGURE 3-37 Bilateral renal artery stenosis and right renal artery stent placement. A, A 78-year-old female with resistant hypertension presented for evaluation. On examination, an abdominal bruit was auscultated. Noninvasive imaging diagnosed bilateral renal artery stenosis. Therefore, the patient underwent renal angiography. Using a pigtail catheter, via the right femoral artery, an abdominal aortic angiogram was performed. This confirmed bilateral renal artery stenosis, right more severe than the left. **B,** The patient underwent stent placement to the right renal artery with successful reduction of the lesion.

FIGURE 3-38 Left internal carotid artery stenosis and stent placement with residual stenosis. A, A 71-year-old female presented with amaurosis fugax of the left eye. Noninvasive evaluation was consistent with significant left carotid stenosis. At angiography, a lesion was noted in the proximal segment of the left internal carotid artery. **B,** Angiogram obtained after intervention. A tapered stent has been deployed into the left distal common carotid artery crossing into the proximal internal carotid artery. Note that there is residual stenosis present, and the ostium of the external carotid artery is now much narrower compared to the pre-intervention angiogram.

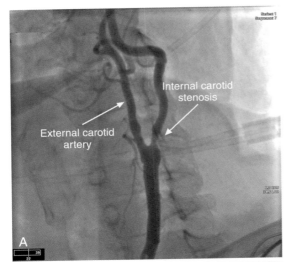

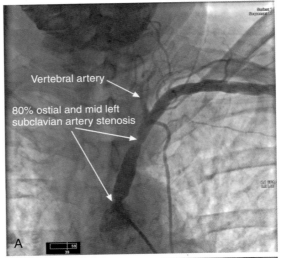

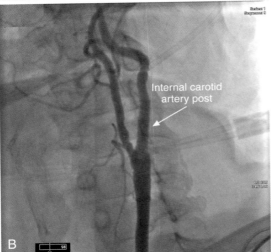

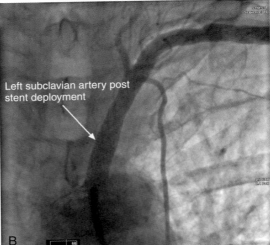

FIGURE 3-39 Left internal carotid artery stenosis and stent placement. A, A 75-year-old female presented for evaluation several weeks after an episode of transient slurring of her speech. Noninvasive imaging was consistent with severe left internal carotid artery stenosis. This angiogram of the left carotid artery was obtained in the LAO projection. This orientation separates the origins of the internal and external carotid arteries. A significant stenosis at the origin of the left internal carotid artery is apparent. **B,** A tapered stent was deployed across the lesion. Final angiograms show no evidence of residual stenosis.

FIGURE 3-40 Left subclavian stenosis and stent placement. A, An 80-year-old female presented with complaints of weakness, dizziness, and left arm discomfort with use of that arm. Examination suggested left subclavian stenosis. An angiogram was obtained using a Judkins right catheter placed at the origin of the left subclavian artery. Note the stenoses at the ostium and mid segment of the left subclavian artery. The vertebral artery is also visualized. On motion angiography, biphasic flow was present within the vertebral artery indicating that the lesions were significant and compromising flow to the arm. **B,** This image was obtained after a stent was successfully placed across both lesions within the left subclavian artery. In addition, it was noted on motion angiography that a normal flow pattern was restored within the vertebral artery.

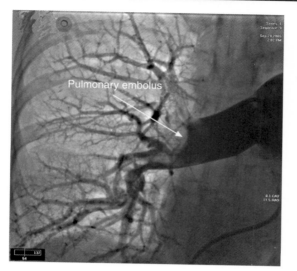

FIGURE 3-41 Right pulmonary artery embolus.
A selective right pulmonary artery angiogram is shown here. Note the large filling defect present in the distal portion of the artery. This is a large pulmonary embolus. Pulmonary angiography remains the gold standard for diagnosis of pulmonary emboli. Nowadays, however, it is rarely performed. More commonly, a CT scan of the chest with contrast or a V/Q scan is obtained in a patient with symptoms suggestive of pulmonary embolus.

CARDIOVASCULAR COMPUTED TOMOGRAPHY

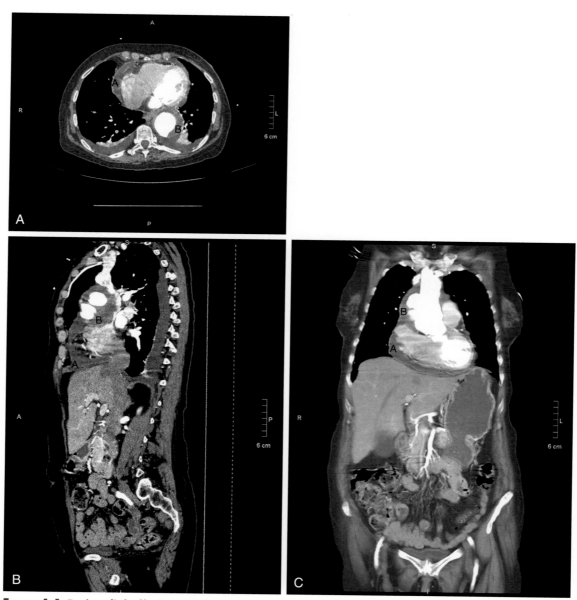

FIGURE 4-1 Pericardial effusion. Axial image from contrast-enhanced CT (**A**) with sagittal (**B**) and coronal (**C**) reconstructions. All of the images demonstrate moderate pericardial fluid (A). This fluid also extends superiorly around the great vessels and tracks inferior around the descending thoracic aorta (B).

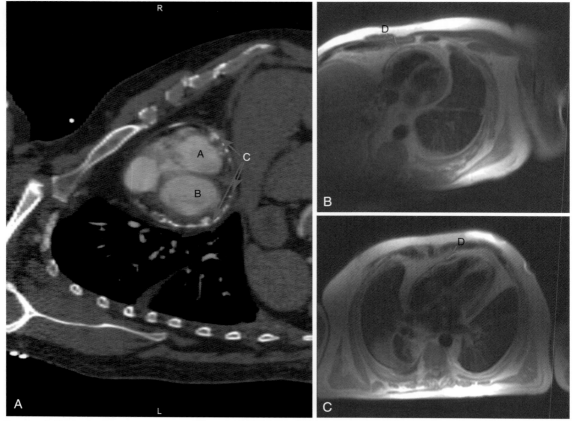

FIGURE 4-2 **Pericarditis. A,** A single short-axis postcontrast CT view of the heart demonstrates extensive calcification (C) of the pericardium adjacent to the right (A) and left (B) ventricles. Short-axis (**B**) and horizontal long-axis (**C**) postcontrast MRI views of the heart demonstrate enhancement of the pericardium (D), especially around the right ventricular wall.

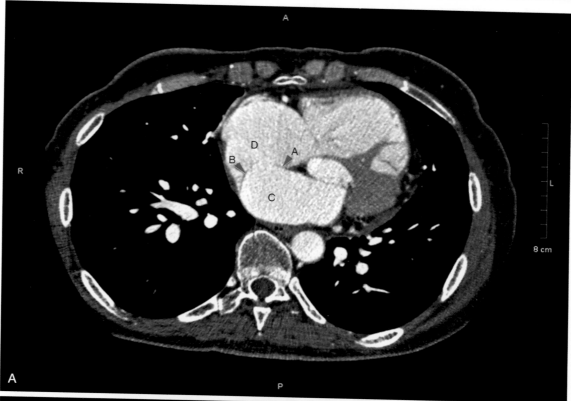

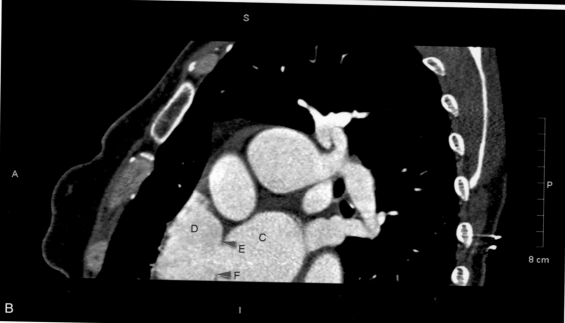

FIGURE 4-3 Atrial septal defect. A gated axial postcontrast-enhanced CT (**A**) with short-axis reconstruction (**B**) demonstrates a large ASD between the left (C) and right (D) atria. The residual anterior (A) and posterior (B) portions of the septum can be seen on the axial image. The short-axis image demonstrates the superior (E) and inferior (F) portions of the atrial septum. A gated cardiac MRI may demonstrate the direction of flow.

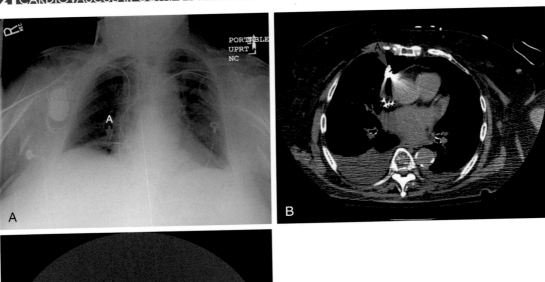

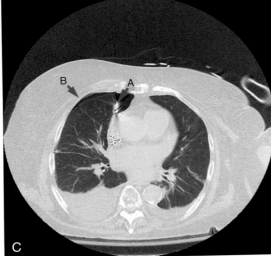

FIGURE 4-4 Pacer lead perforation. Frontal chest x-ray (**A**) and axial noncontrast chest CT in mediastinal (**B**) and lung (**C**) windows. **A,** The chest x-ray demonstrates two sets of pacer leads with an atrial lead (A) that does not appear to be over the cardiac silhouette. **B,** Chest CT then clearly demonstrates that the atrial lead has perforated the anterior right atrial wall (A). **C,** The lung windows demonstrate a small anterior pneumothorax (B), not visible on the chest x-ray.

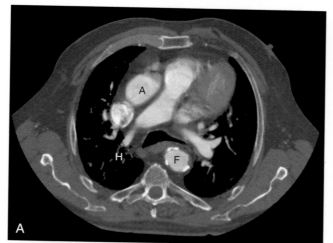

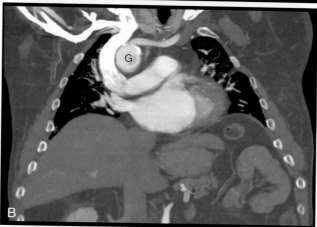

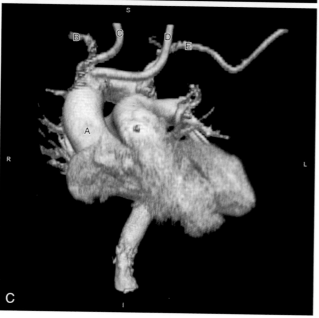

FIGURE 4-5 Right-sided arch. Axial postcontrast-enhanced CT (**A**) with MIP coronal reconstruction (**B**) and a 3D view (**C**). A right-sided ascending aorta (A) is seen with a right-sided aortic arch (G) that passes posterior to the esophagus and trachea (H). Aberrant origin of the right carotid artery (C) is present but is not well visualized on this exam. The right subclavian (B) and left carotid (D) arteries are grossly unremarkable. The origin of the left subclavian artery (E) is more distal arising from the aortic arch. The aorta descends on the left side of the spine (F).

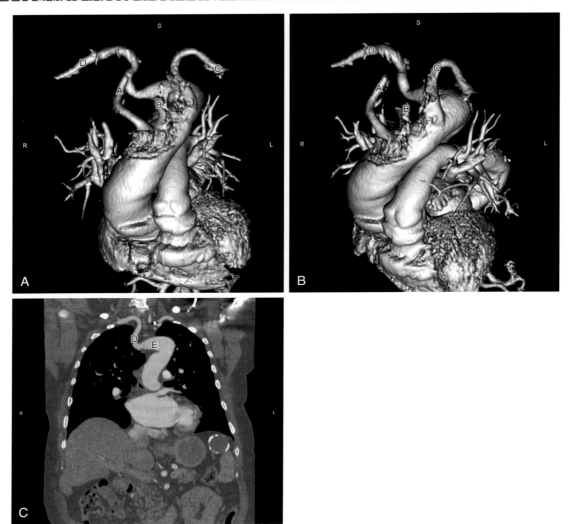

FIGURE 4-6 Anomalous great vessels. Contrast-enhanced CT with 3D MIP views (**A** and **B**) and coronal reconstruction (**C**). The anomalous order of great vessels as they originate from the aortic arch is right carotid artery (A), left carotid artery (B), left subclavian artery (C), and finally right subclavian artery (D). The anomalous right subclavian artery passes behind the esophagus. The dilated origin of the right subclavian artery is called the diverticulum of Kommerell (E).

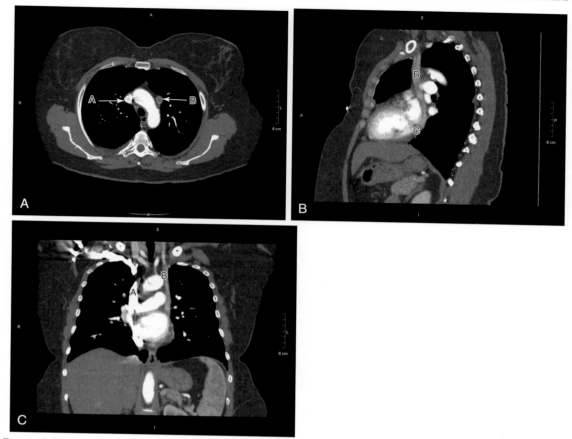

FIGURE 4-7 Persistent left SVC. Axial contrast-enhanced CT (**A**) with sagittal (**B**) and coronal (**C**) reconstructions. **A,** The axial image shows a densely contrast filled right SVC (A) with less dense contrast in the left SVC (B). **B** and **C,** The sagittal and coronal views demonstrate the course of the left SVC draining into the coronary sinus (C). The incidence of a persistent left SVC is 0.3%.

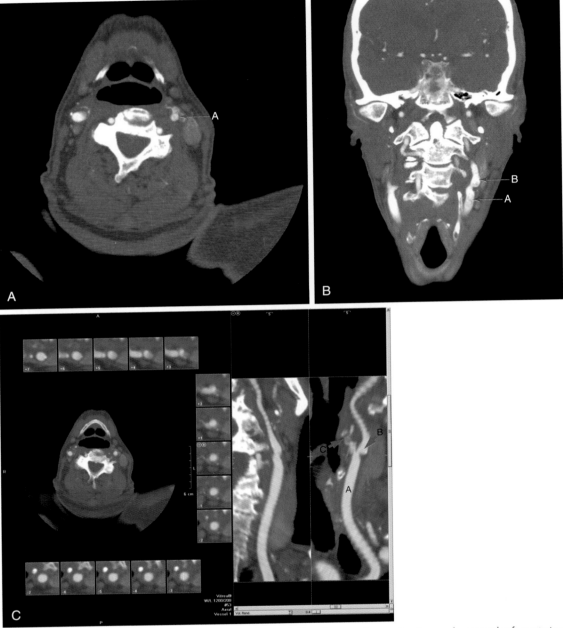

FIGURE 4-8 Carotid stenosis. Axial postcontrast-enhanced CT with coronal reconstruction and a curved reformat view. The coronal image (**B**) demonstrates a tortuous left common carotid artery (A) with a narrowing of the proximal left internal carotid artery (B) at its origin. The full extent of the stenosis is more clearly visualized on the curved reformat view. In addition, note the stenosis present in the proximal left external carotid artery (C).

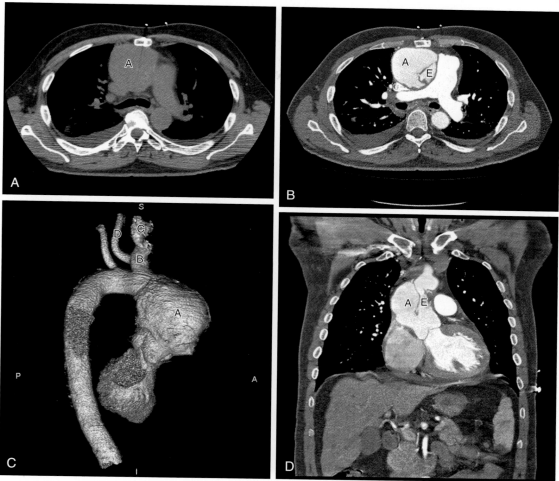

FIGURE 4-9 Ascending aortic aneurysm. Axial precontrast (**A**) and postcontrast (**B**) enhanced CT with 3D MIP view (**C**) and coronal reconstruction (**D**). Precontrast images demonstrate no evidence of an intramural hemorrhage, but the postcontrast image demonstrates a right lateral aneurysm (not dissection) (A). The coronal postcontrast image shows compression of the ascending aorta (E) by the ascending aortic aneurysm. The ascending location is also demonstrated on the 3D MIP reconstruction, along with the incidental finding of a bovine arch with right innominate artery (C) and left carotid artery (D) sharing a common origin (B).

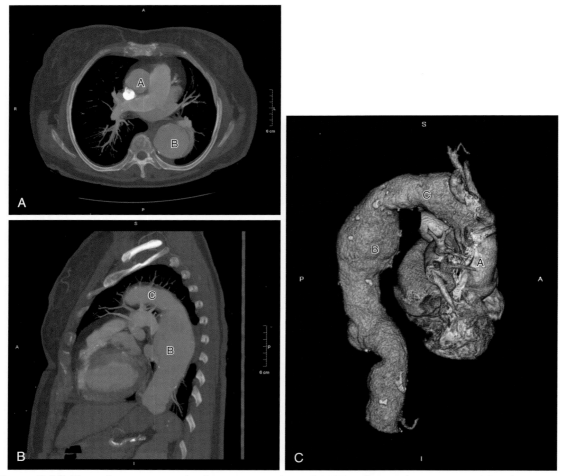

FIGURE 4-10 Thoracic aneurysm. Axial postcontrast enhanced CT (**A**) with sagittal reconstruction (**B**) and a 3D view (**C**). The axial and 3D views demonstrate a normal ascending aorta (A) and the descending thoracic aortic aneurysm (B) within the thorax. The sagittal view demonstrates a normal aortic arch (C) with the midthoracic aortic aneurysm (B).

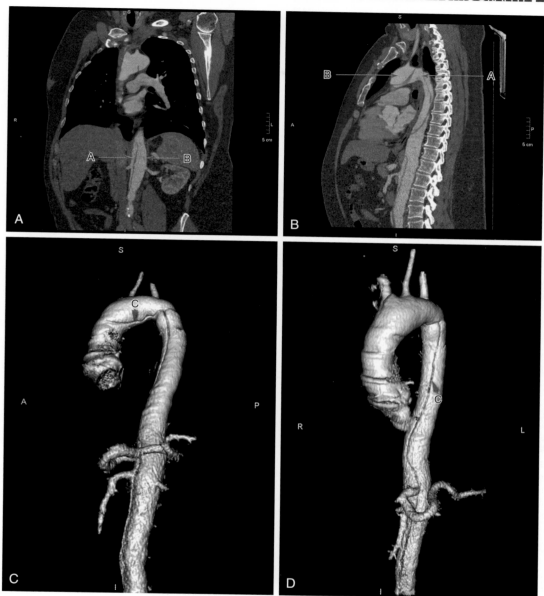

FIGURE 4-11 Stanford type A aortic dissection. Postcontrast enhanced CT with coronal (**A**) and sagittal (**B**) reconstructions with 3D reconstructions (**C** and **D**). The coronal and sagittal reconstructions demonstrate the dissection with contrast filling both the true (A) and false (B) lumens throughout the entirety of the dissection. The 3D reconstructions show the dissection (C) starting in the ascending aorta and continuing into the abdominal aorta.

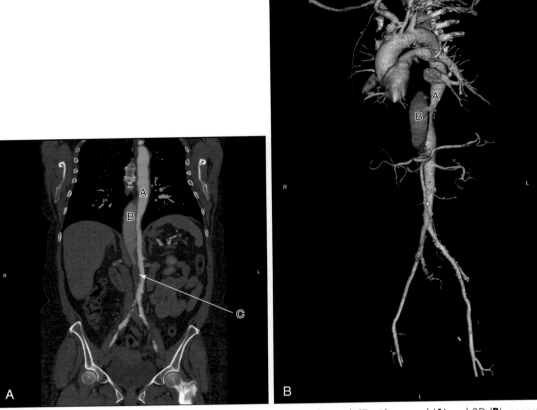

FIGURE 4-12 Stanford type B aortic dissection. Postcontrast enhanced CT with coronal (**A**) and 3D (**B**) reconstructions. The coronal reconstruction demonstrates dense contrast filling the true lumen of a descending aortic dissection (A) with compression and flattening of the true lumen by the false lumen (B). The false lumen is partially thrombosed (C), and the contrast visualized within the false lumen is less dense than the true lumen. The dissection is limited to the aorta distal to the left subclavian artery and is therefore classified as a Stanford type B dissection.

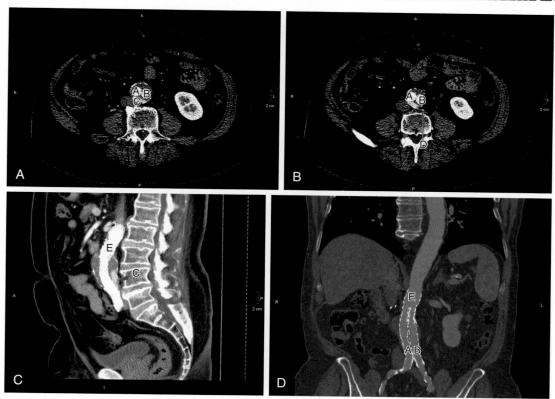

FIGURE 4-13 Type II endoleak. Axial postcontrast-enhanced CT images (**A** and **B**) with sagittal (**C**) and coronal (**D**) reconstructions. The coronal view demonstrates a stent graft in the distal abdominal aorta (E) that extends into the right (A) and left (B) iliac arteries. The sagittal view demonstrates contrast within the stent graft; however, contrast is also present within the portion of the aortic aneurysm that is supposed to be excluded by the stent graft (C). The axial images demonstrate that a lumbar artery (D) with reversed flow is the source of the contrast leak. This is classified as a type II endoleak. (For reference, see White GH, May J, Waugh RC, et al. Type III and type IV endoleak: toward a complete definition of blood flow in the sac after endoluminal AAA repair. *J Endovasc Surg* 1998;5:305–309.)

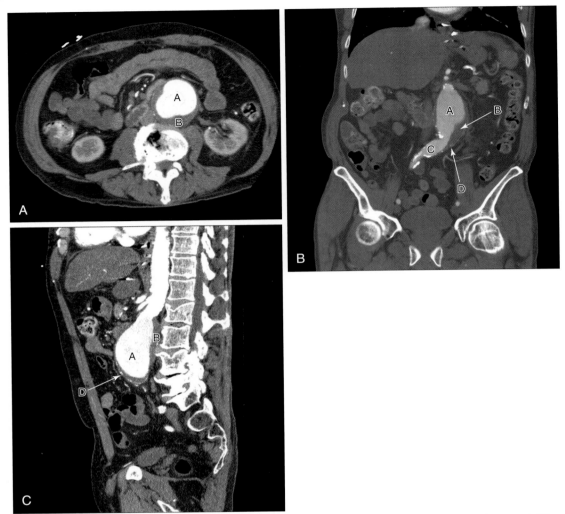

Figure 4-14 Abdominal aortic aneurysm. Axial image from a contrast-enhanced CT (**A**) with coronal (**B**) and sagittal (**C**) reconstructions. The images demonstrate contrast within an AAA (>5 cm) (A). Mural thrombus (B) can be seen between the contrast and the aortic wall, which contains calcium (D). The coronal image demonstrates the aneurysm extending into the right common iliac artery (C). Measurement of the aneurysm, in evaluating for possible treatment, should include the portion containing contrast and the portion with the thrombus (A and B).

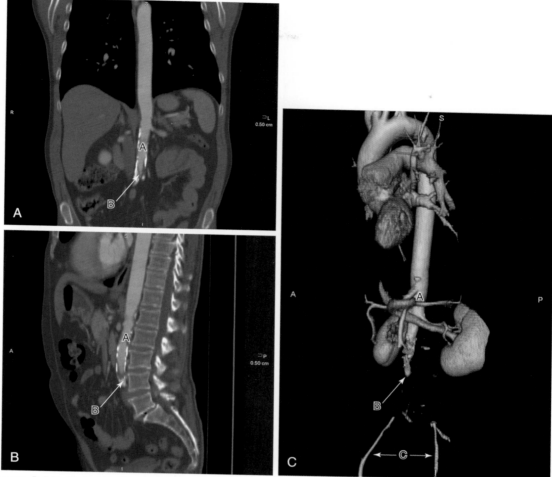

FIGURE 4-15 Abdominal aortic occlusion. A contrast-enhanced CT with coronal (**A**) and sagittal (**B**) reconstructions and 3D MIP view (**C**). Contrast is seen within the abdominal aorta (A) to just above the bifurcation of the iliac arteries, at which level there is complete thrombosis (B) of the distal aorta and the common iliac arteries. Note the calcification within the aortic wall at this site. The 3D reconstructions demonstrate reconstitution of the bilateral femoral arteries from collaterals (C). This is a chronic occlusion with enlargement of the collateral vessels (not seen on these images) to reconstitute the femoral arteries.

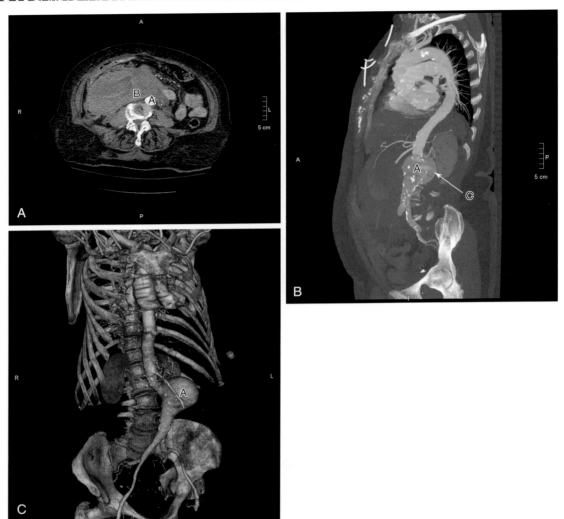

FIGURE 4-16 Ruptured AAA. Axial postcontrast-enhanced CT (**A**) with sagittal reconstruction (**B**) and a 3D MIP view (**C**). The sagittal reconstruction demonstrates a large infrarenal AAA (A) with contrast (C) outside the calcified aorta. The 3D view demonstrates the large size of the AAA. The axial postcontrast image demonstrates a large intra-abdominal hematoma (B) from the ruptured aneurysm.

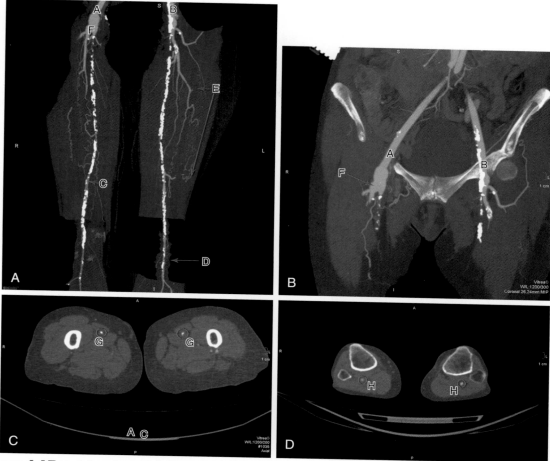

FIGURE 4-17 Peripheral arterial disease. Coronal MIP views of the femoral vessels (**A**) and bilateral pelvic vessels (**B**), as well as contrasted axial midthigh (**C**) and distal thigh (**D**) CT images. The femoral MIP views demonstrate the distal portions of right (A) and left (B) femoral artery grafts as well as absent proximal SFAs and patent distal bilateral SFAs and popliteal arteries (C and D). Extensive collateral vessels with a corkscrew appearance are present in the thighs (E) that reconstitute the distal vessels. The coronal MIP image of the pelvis demonstrates the bilateral grafts (A and B) and an incidental pseudoaneurysm at the distal aspect of the right graft (F). On the axial images of the midthigh, there is no contrast in the bilateral SFAs. Only calcium (G) is noted. Contrast is seen in the reconstituted bilateral popliteal arteries in the distal thighs (H).

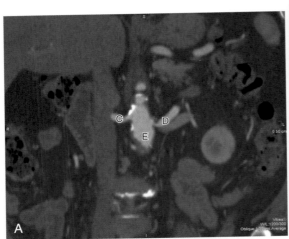

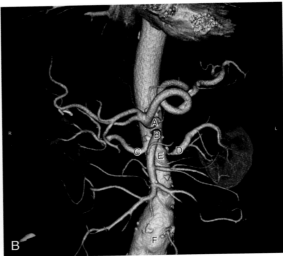

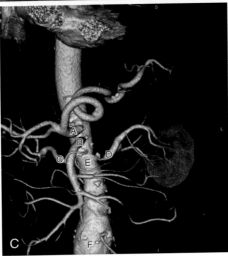

Figure 4-18 Renal artery stenosis. Coronal reconstruction of postcontrast abdominal CT (**A**) with AP (**B**) and oblique (**C**) views of 3D images of the abdominal aorta and branching vessels. The coronal image shows a portion of the abdominal aorta (E) with the right (C) and left (D) renal arteries. A severe stenosis of the proximal left renal artery is present. The 3D images show the abdominal aorta with a small infrarenal aneurysm (F). The celiac (A) and superior mesenteric (B) arteries are also labeled for reference. Calcified plaque is present at the origin of the right renal artery, but there is no significant stenosis.

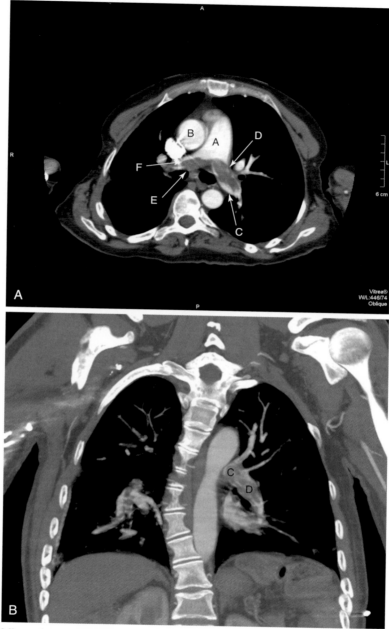

FIGURE 4-19 Saddle pulmonary embolism. Axial postcontrast-enhanced CT (**A**) with coronal reconstruction (**B**). The filling defect in the main pulmonary artery (A) extends into the right and left pulmonary arteries. The axial image demonstrates that contrast is present within the patent portion of the left pulmonary artery (C). The filling defect represents the thrombus (D). The right pulmonary artery has thrombosed (E) and patent (F) portions. The thrombus can be seen extending from the left pulmonary artery into the left lower pulmonary artery on the coronal reformat. The aorta (B) is also labeled for reference.

ADULT CARDIAC MR CASES

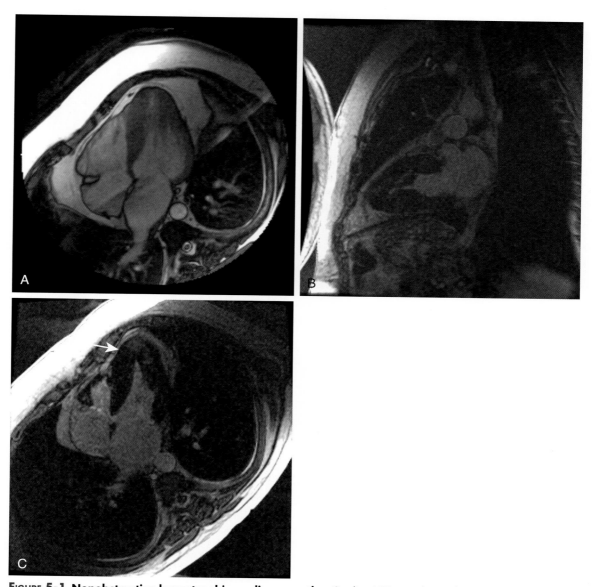

FIGURE 5-1 Nonobstructive hypertrophic cardiomyopathy. Cardiac MRI is used to evaluate the severity and location of hypertrophy and fibrosis in HCM. Cine imaging is used to evaluate dynamic outflow tract obstruction from the systolic anterior motion of the anterior mitral valve leaflet.

Cardiac MRI was performed to evaluate a 20-year-old white male presenting with worsening exertional dyspnea and near-syncope. His brother died suddenly at age 23. An echocardiogram showed symmetric hypertrophy without evidence of a dynamic outflow tract obstruction. **A,** The horizontal WB long-axis image shows diffuse hypertrophic changes of the LV walls. Postcontrast vertical (**B**) and horizontal (**C**) long-axis images demonstrate areas of hyperenhancement (*arrow*) from myocardial fibrosis at the cardiac apex. This fibrosis is associated with increased risk of heart failure and sudden death.

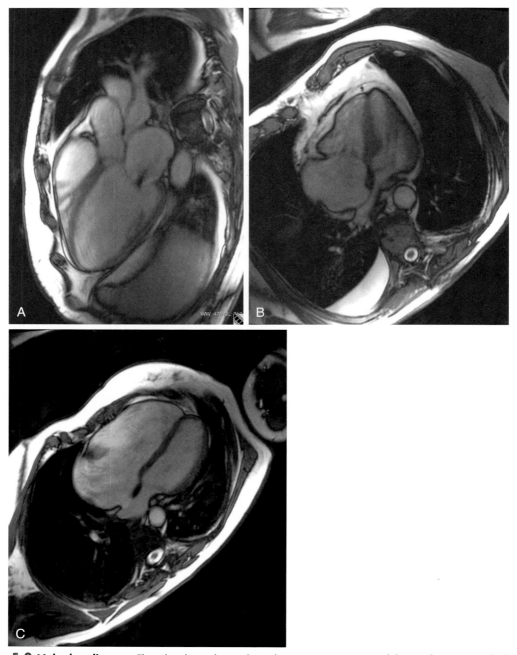

FIGURE 5-2 Valvular disease. Though echocardiography is the primary imaging modality used to assess valvular structures, regurgitation, and stenosis, cardiac MRI is useful in patients with suboptimal echocardiographic images. Valve leaflet thickness and mobility can be assessed. In addition, quantification of valvular regurgitation may be completed using phase and volumetric techniques. **A,** Mitral regurgitation. A 72-year-old African American male with longstanding hypertension presented with progressive heart failure. On cardiac MRI, this WB LV inflow view demonstrates an enlarged LV with significant mitral regurgitation, represented by the black jet in the white blood extending from the valve into the left atrium. **B,** Tricuspid stenosis. A 30-year-old female presented with symptoms of progressive right heart failure, increasing abdominal pain, ascites, and lower extremity edema over the past few months. Cardiac MRI demonstrated a normal RV but thickened tricuspid valve leaflets. The right atrium is markedly enlarged, and an incidental right pleural effusion can be seen on this WB horizontal long-axis view. **C,** Ebstein anomaly. Cardiac MRI demonstrates a markedly enlarged right atrium and RV on this WB horizontal long-axis view. The tricuspid valve leaflets are not well visualized. The leftward bowing of the atrial septum is consistent with increased right-sided pressures. The patient was a 70-year-old female who presented with a vague history of cardiac murmur and 6-month history of abdominal swelling and lower extremity edema. Echocardiography demonstrated inferior displacement of the septal leaflet of the tricuspid valve, a dilated right atrium and RV, and severe tricuspid regurgitation consistent with Ebstein anomaly.

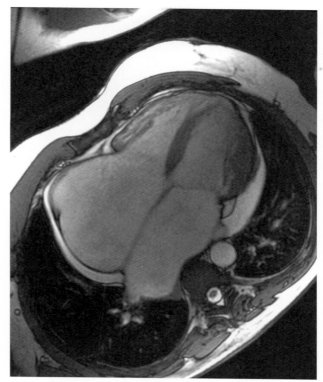

FIGURE 5-3 Restrictive cardiomyopathy. WB horizontal long-axis image obtained from a 60-year-old male whot had felt poorly for several years but had become more dyspneic over the past 3 months. The patient's history includes Hodgkin lymphoma as a teenager with mantle radiation. Cardiac MRI, completed to help determine if the patient had restrictive cardiomyopathy versus constrictive pericarditis, demonstrated normal LV and RV cavity sizes and systolic function. Both left and right atria are massively enlarged. No significant valvular regurgitation was seen. The pericardium is of normal thickness. The patient was diagnosed with restrictive cardiomyopathy.

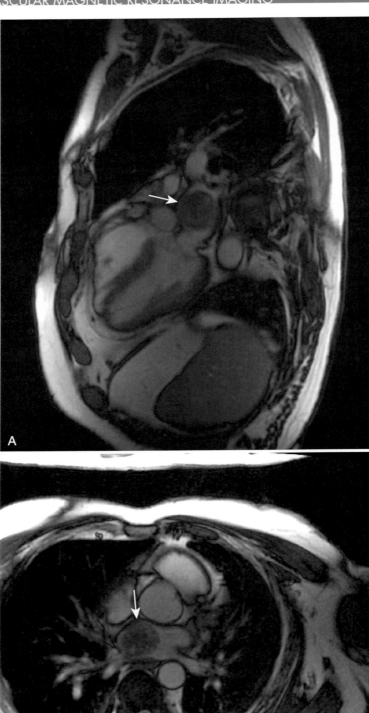

FIGURE 5-4 Left atrial myxoma. A 45-year-old Native American male evaluated for a several-month history of night sweats and several episodes of positional near-syncope, particularly when he goes bowling. TTE had demonstrated a left atrial mass, and cardiac MRI confirmed that the large left atrial mass occupying the superior portion of the left atrium was a myxoma (*arrows*). The mass appears homogeneous and smooth with a capsule. WB vertical long-axis (**A**) and axial (**B**) images demonstrate the left atrial myxoma. Often, contrast is administered to help differentiate cardiac masses. For example, lymphomas are usually markedly enhancing, whereas myxomas usually do not significantly enhance.

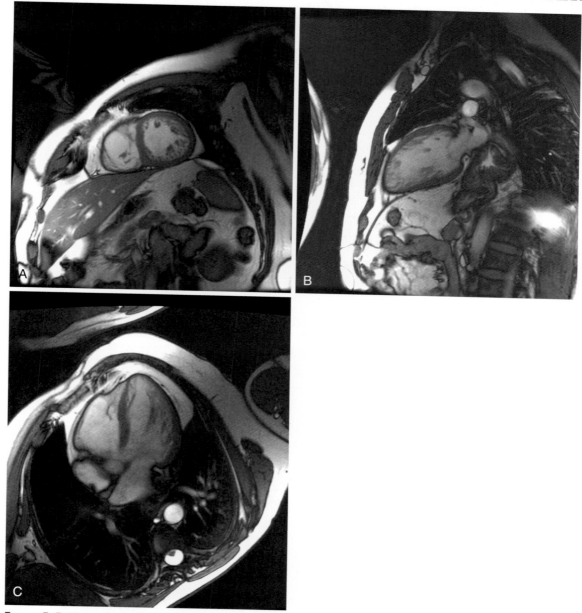

FIGURE 5-5 Noncompaction cardiomyopathy. A 35-year-old white female presented with heart failure and no prior cardiac history. TTE was technically challenging, but demonstrated a normal LV size with prominent trabeculations at the apex. WB T2-weighted images in short-axis (**A**), vertical long-axis (**B**), and horizontal long-axis (**C**) demonstrate a thickened LV wall secondary to thickened trabeculations. Blood is clearly viewed within the thick trabeculations. This patient was diagnosed with noncompaction cardiomyopathy.

FIGURE 5-6 Anomalous LCA. A 20-year-old African American female presented with recurrent exertional chest pain. This fat-suppressed T2-weighted axial image reveals an abnormal course of the LCA (*arrow*) between the aorta and main PA trunk. This is a known risk factor for sudden cardiac death in young adults during exercise. The LCA may be compressed between the aorta and PA during episodes of increased cardiac output.

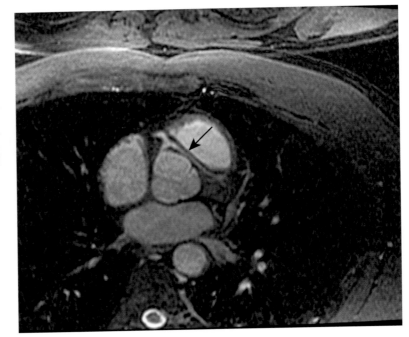

FIGURE 5-7 Cor triatriatum sinistrum. A 27-year-old white male presented with dyspnea and a heart murmur. The T1-weighted axial cardiac MRI shown here demonstrates cor triatriatum sinistrum. The left atrium is partitioned into two segments by a fibromuscular membrane (*arrow*). The posterosuperior portion usually receives the pulmonary venous return, and the anteroinferior portion contains the left atrial appendage and mitral valve. In this image, the LV appears normal in size. The RV is prominent with low normal function on cine imaging. Depending on the presence and size of the communication(s) present, pulmonary hypertension may develop secondary to obstruction of pulmonary venous flow. In symptomatic patients, the membrane can be surgically resected. There are several theories of development of cor triatriatum sinistrum, including malincorporation, malseptation, and entrapment.

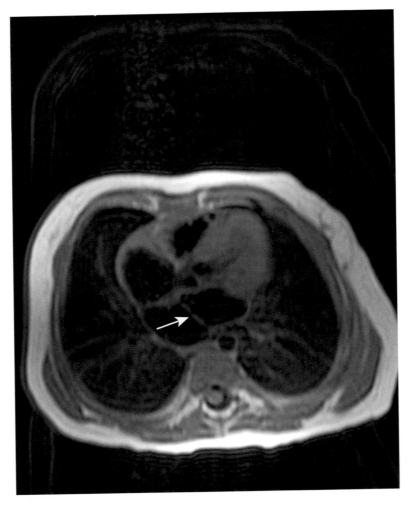

ADULT CONGENITAL MR CASES

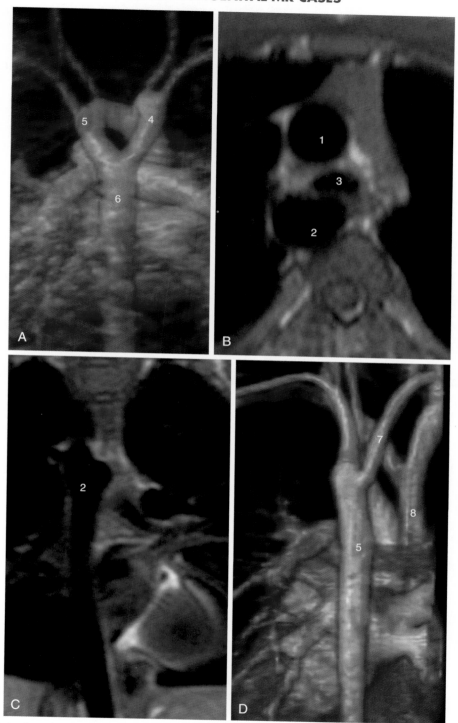

FIGURE 5-8 Aortic arch anomalies can occasionally escape detection until adulthood if symptoms are mild. **A,** A double aortic arch that forms a vascular ring (posterior view of surface-rendered image). Black blood axial (**B**) and coronal (**C**) images of a right aortic arch with a Kommerell diverticulum and mirror image branching of the brachiocephalic vessels. This anomaly also forms a vascular ring. Kommerell diverticulum is the bulb-like dilatation of the distal origin of the left subclavian artery from the descending thoracic aorta. **D,** A left aortic arch with retro-esophageal right subclavian artery. This is not a vascular ring but may cause mild dysphagia. 1, Ascending aorta; 2, descending aorta, with Kommerell diverticulum in part **C**; 3, trachea at bifurcation; 4, right arch; 5, left arch; 6, descending aorta; 7, anomalous right subclavian artery; 8, SVC.

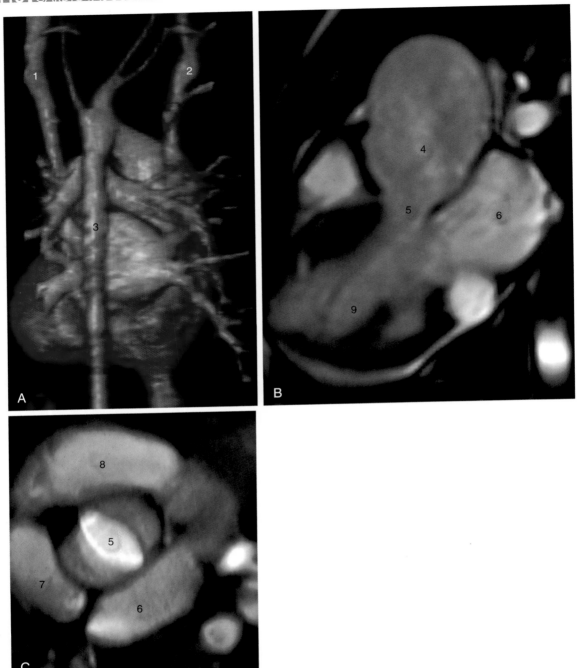

FIGURE 5-9 Associated defects of aortic arch anomalies should always be potentially investigated. **A,** A surface-rendered posterior view of a patient who has previously undergone subclavian flap repair of coarctation. Note absence of a left sub-clavian artery and bilateral SVC. **B,** In this three-chamber view, an enlarged aortic root and ascending aortic aneurysm are apparent. **C,** The aortic valve was determined to be bicuspid on short-axis imaging. Coarctation of the aorta is commonly associated with bicuspid aortic valve. 1, Left SVC; 2, right SVC; 3, descending aorta; 4, aortic root enlargement; 5, bicuspid aortic valve; 6, left atrium; 7, right atrium; 8, RV; 9, LV.

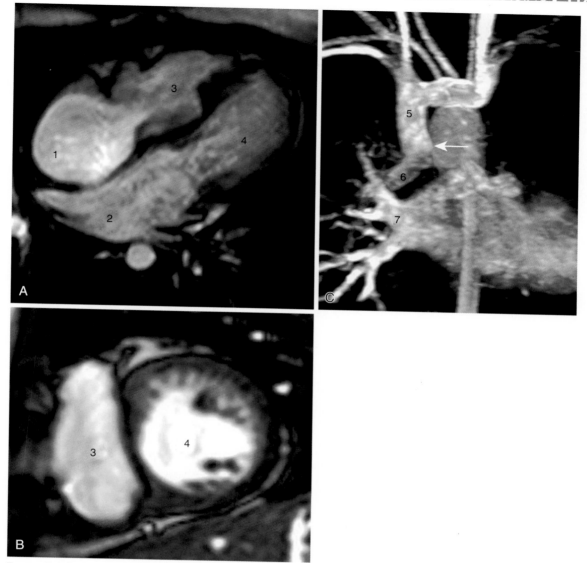

FIGURE 5-10 When a child is born with inadequate ventricle or AV valve size, a 1½ ventricle repair may be completed. Horizontal (**A**) and short-axis (**B**) images of the cardiac chambers. In this patient, the RV was dysfunctional and the right atrium was enlarged. Therefore, the patient underwent a Glenn operation, which allows blood to flow passively from the SVC to the PAs (*arrow*). The pulmonary arteries are confluent in this patient; however, secondary to asymmetric gadolinium enhancement, part **C** lends the impression of a classic unidirectional Glenn shunt, instead of a bidirectional Glenn shunt. After the Glenn shunt, the RV only receives IVC flow and pumps this blood through the pulmonary artery. 1, Right atrium; 2, left atrium; 3, RV; 4, LV; 5, SVC; 6, right PA; 7, right pulmonary veins.

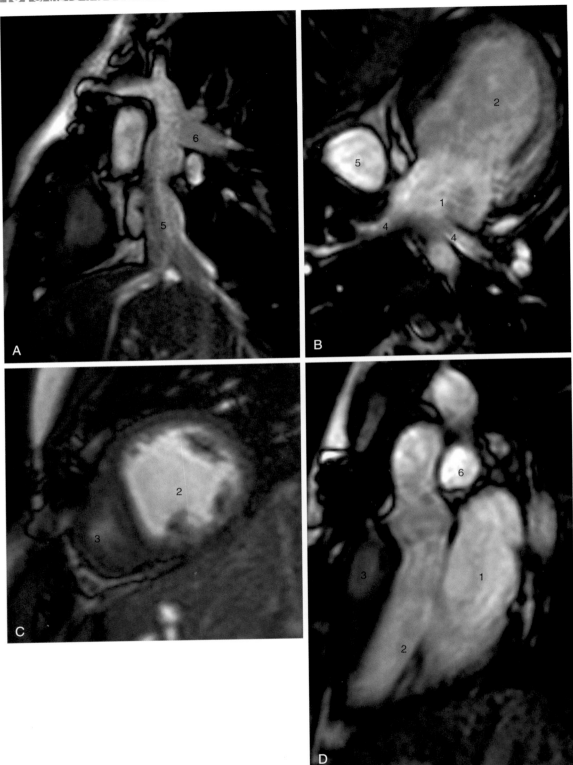

FIGURE 5-11 A patient with tricuspid atresia and a tiny RV who has undergone a staged palliation culminating in a Fontan procedure. **A,** The Fontan procedure results in venous blood from both the SVC and IVC passively flowing to the pulmonary circulation, bypassing a pumping chamber. Horizontal long-axis (**B**), short-axis (**C**), and three-chamber (**D**) images of the functional single ventricle that pumps to the systemic circulation. The TV is absent and the RV is hypoplastic and hypertrophied. 1, Left atrium; 2, LV; 3, hypoplastic/hypertrophied RV; 4, pulmonary veins; 5, Fontan pathway; 6, PAs.

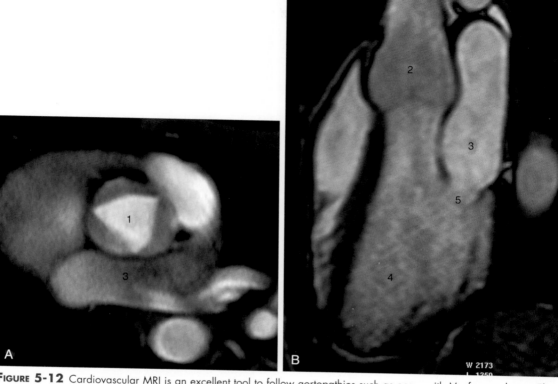

FIGURE 5-12 Cardiovascular MRI is an excellent tool to follow aortopathies such as occur with Marfan syndrome. These WB short-axis (**A**) and three-chamber (**B**) images depict a trileaflet aortic valve with aortic root dilation. 1, Aortic valve in systole; 2, aortic root; 3, left atrium; 4, LV; 5, mitral valve.

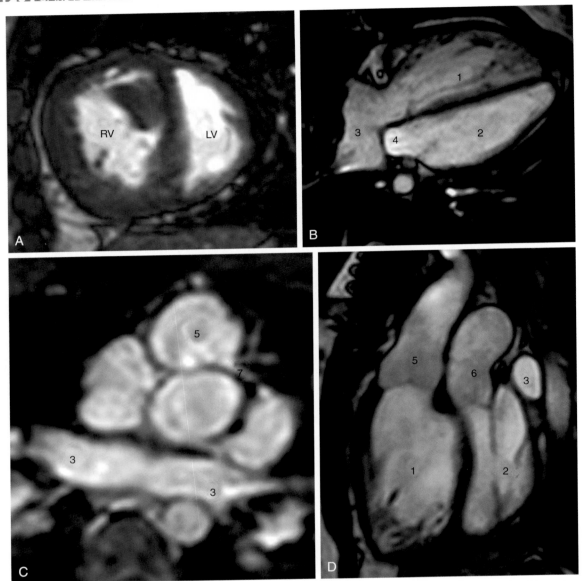

FIGURE 5-13 Many patients born with D-transposition before the late 1980s underwent surgical repair with a Mustard or Senning operation. This operation leaves the great vessels transposed and places the RV as the systemic pump. This operation involves placing an intra-atrial baffle to direct pulmonary venous return to the systemic RV and systemic venous blood to the subpulmonary LV. **A,** Short-axis view of the ventricles showing RV enlargement, hypertrophy, and flattening of the septum. **B,** Horizontal long-axis image demonstrating the anterior RV receiving flow via the pulmonary views pathway. **C,** Axial (short-axis) image of pulmonary venous pathway. **D,** Sagittal view of the cardiac chambers. Note the RV is the systemic pumping chamber connected to the aorta. It is severely enlarged and hypertrophied. The LV is connected to the pulmonary artery. Note the absence of hypertrophy of this chamber's walls. 1, RV; 2, LV; 3, pulmonary venous pathway; 4, systemic venous pathway; 5, aorta (anterior); 6, PA (posterior); 7, LCA.

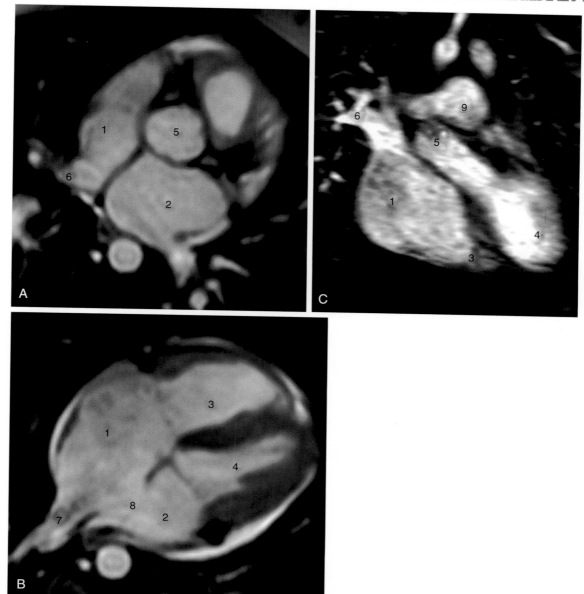

FIGURE 5-14 ASDs are occasionally associated with PAPVR. Both result in right-sided volume overload and RV enlargement. **A,** Paraxial image demonstrating the RUPV draining into the right atrium. **B,** Horizontal long-axis (four-chamber) image showing the right lower pulmonary vein emptying into a massively enlarged right atrium. A large secundum ASD is present. Also note the biventricular hypertrophy and RV cavity dilatation. Anomalous pulmonary venous drainage is relatively rare in patients with secundum ASDs. However, sinus venosus ASDs are nearly always associated with PAPVR, most commonly involving the RUPV, as shown in part **C**. In this oblique coronal view, the RUPV is draining into a severely enlarged right atrium. 1, Right atrium; 2, left atrium; 3, RV; 4, LV; 5, aorta; 6, right upper pulmonary vein; 7, right lower pulmonary vein; 8, ASD; 9, PA.

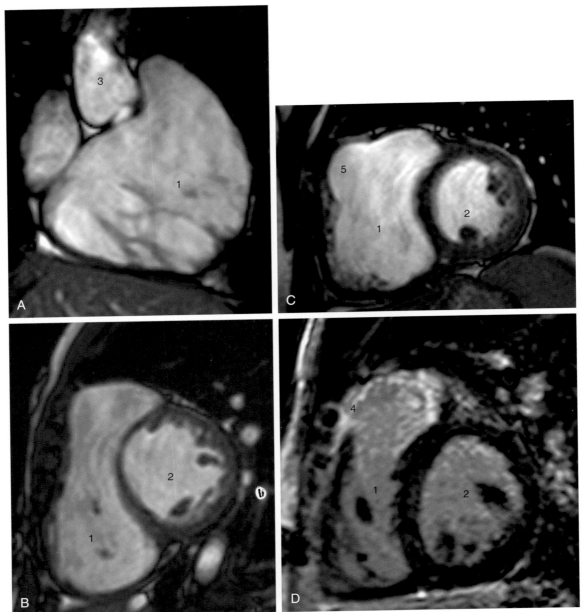

FIGURE 5-15 Postoperative evaluation of tetralogy of Fallot frequently involves the use of cardiac MRI. After transannular repair of the RVOT, patients may develop significant RV pathology, including enlargement, fibrosis, poor function, or areas of dyskinesis. MRI can also be used to quantify flow and calculate a regurgitant fraction. This data is important in decision making for replacement of the pulmonary valve. **A,** WB paracoronal image demonstrating marked RV enlargement in a patient with a history of repair for tetralogy of Fallot. **B** and **C,** Short-axis images from different patients with tetralogy of Fallot repairs showing RV enlargement. The patient in part **C** also has developed aneurismal dilatation of the RVOT. **D,** Delayed enhancement short-axis image showing fibrosis in the RV outflow region. 1, RV; 2, LV; 3, aorta; 4, delayed enhancement; 5, RVOT aneurysm.

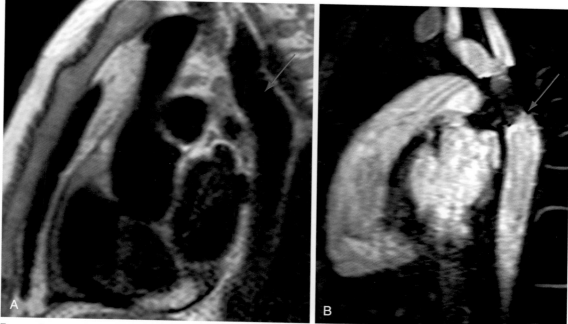

FIGURE 5-16 Aortic coarctation can be treated surgically or in older children and adults by transcatheter therapy. Aortic coarctation beyond the early childhood years is frequently treated with endovascular stent placement. Current stents (*arrows*) may cause significant signal void on WB images; however, useful information can be obtained using black blood images. Sagittal black blood (**A**) and white blood (**B**) images in a patient after endovascular treatment of aortic coarctation. Note the signal void caused by the stent on the WB image. Cardiac MRI/MRA is the modality of choice to longitudinally follow repaired coarctations; the major concerns are recurrent coarctation and aneurysm formation.

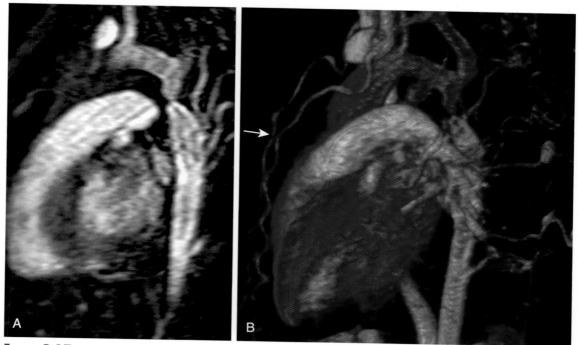

FIGURE 5-17 Native coarctation presents with upper extremity hypertension. In an older child or young adult extensive aortic collaterals are often present with enlargement of vessels proximal to the obstruction such as internal mammary arteries. Aortic coarctation is frequently associated with relative hypoplasia of the transverse aortic arch. **A,** Gadolinium-enhanced MRA in the sagittal plane. **B,** Surface-rendered image viewed from the left chest perspective. Note the large internal mammary arteries (*arrows*) and hypoplasia of the transverse arch just before the coarctation. If left untreated, significant transverse arch hypoplasia may be associated with right arm and cerebral circulation hypertension.

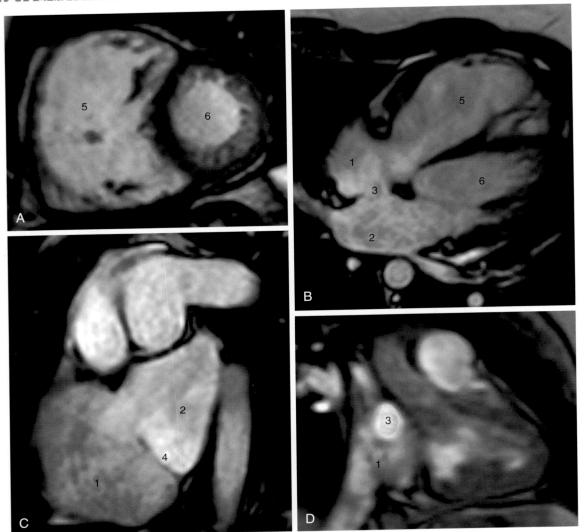

FIGURE 5-18 Ostium secundum ASD can sometimes escape detection until adulthood. Short-axis (**A**) and horizontal long-axis (**B**) images demonstrate the marked RV enlargement characteristically seen in patients with large unrepaired ASDs. In part **B**, the secundum ASD is readily apparent. It can also be used to define tissue rims if consideration of transcatheter intervention is entertained. The inferior or IVC rim is the most difficult to image with echocardiography but is shown well on appropriate MRI images, as noted in part **C. D,** Enface imaging of the atrial septum can provide information about the defect shape and relationship if more than one defect is suspected. 1, Right atrium; 2, left atrium; 3, ASD; 4, inferior rim; 5, RV; 6, LV.

PERIPHERAL VASCULAR MRA CASES

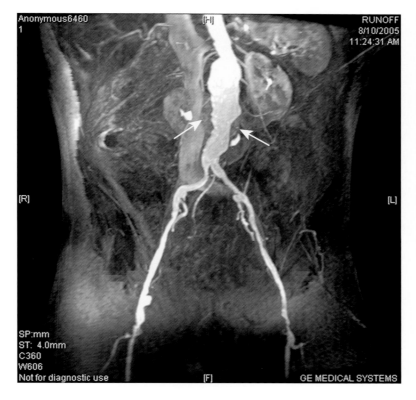

FIGURE 5-19 Infrarenal AAA with bilateral iliac stenoses. A 67-year-old Native American male presented with progressive lower extremity claudication and several necrotic toes. Patient had a history of diabetes, tobacco use, and hyperlipidemia. This single coronal postcontrast MIP MRA shows a large infrarenal AAA with mild circumferential clot (*arrow*). The aneurysm begins 5.6 mm inferior to the main right renal artery and extends 7.8 cm inferiorly to the iliac bifurcation. The maximum diameter is 4.7 cm. There is a 70% stenosis of the proximal right common iliac artery and 40% stenosis of the proximal left common iliac artery.

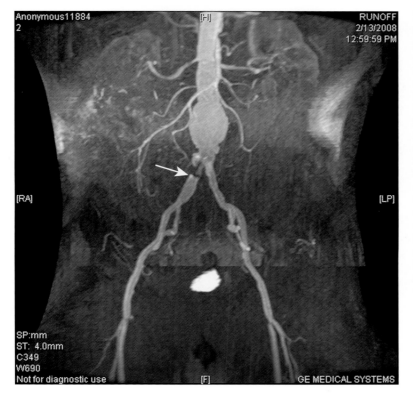

FIGURE 5-20 Infrarenal AAA with right common iliac artery stent. A 72-year-old African American male with known PVD, CAD, hypertension, and diabetes mellitus underwent MRA to further evaluate an AAA found on a duplex study. He had previous right lower extremity claudication and had undergone placement of a right common iliac stent. He had emboli to both feet recently. Single coronal noncontrast MIP MRA shows a large infrarenal AAA that begins 4.1 cm inferior to the origin of the left main renal artery and extends to the iliac bifurcation. The maximum dimension of the AAA is 5.3 cm. Stent artifact is seen in the proximal right common iliac artery (*arrow*); therefore, it is not possible to evaluate the right SFA at the stent location.

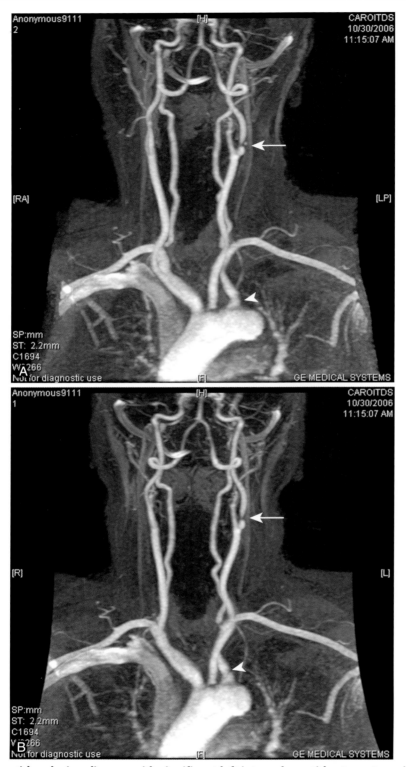

FIGURE 5-21 Carotid occlusive disease with significant left internal carotid artery stenosis: two coronal postcontrast MIP MRA. A 65-year-old white male with hypertension and diabetes presented with transient right hand weakness. Carotid duplex imaging suggested a severe (60% to 79%) stenosis of the proximal left ICA. **A** and **B,** With just slightly different angles, are two coronal postcontrast MIP MRA images showing a 70% to 80% stenosis of the proximal left ICA (*arrows*). There is also a 40% to 50% stenosis of the proximal left subclavian artery (*arrowheads*). In addition, there is a 30% stenosis of the proximal right ICA that is not well-visualized on these images.

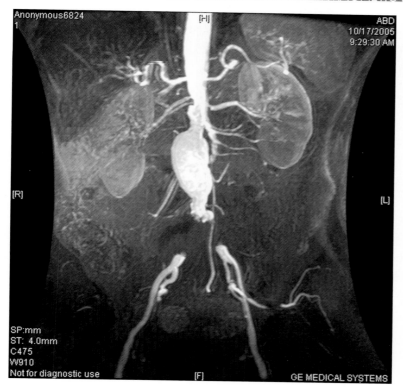

FIGURE 5-22 Infrarenal AAA with occluded distal aorta and bilateral common iliac stents. A 56-year-old Native American male who uses tobacco and has uncontrolled hypertension and diabetes presented with progressive bilateral lower extremity claudication. He has had previous treatment of PVD with stents placed to both common iliac arteries. Abdominal ultrasound diagnosed a large AAA. This coronal postcontrast MIP MRA delineates a large infrarenal AAA arising 3.2 cm below the origins of the renal arteries, extending 6.2 cm distally, and having a maximum dimension of 4 cm in an oblique plane. There is minimal clot within the aneurysm. Note that the aorta distal to the aneurysm is occluded.

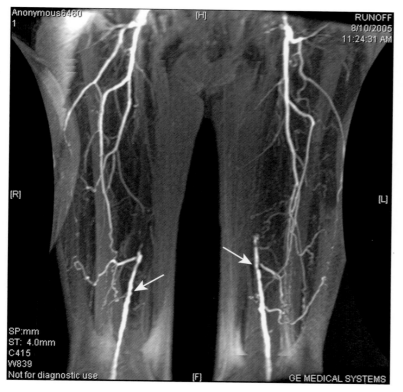

FIGURE 5-23 Bilateral occluded superficial femoral arteries. A 70-year-old white female with hypertension and hyperlipidemia presented with resting and exercise-induced bilateral lower extremity discomfort. She has had progressive claudication over the years, which has become more noticeable over the past few months. Additionally, she now has intermittent rest discomfort. This coronal postcontrast MIP MRA demonstrates 100% occlusion of the proximal right and left SFAs, which reconstitute distally (*arrows*). Corkscrew arteries are present, suggestive of chronic occulusion with collateral development.

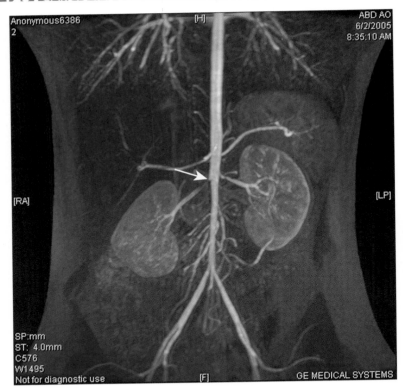

FIGURE 5-24 Right renal artery stenosis with stenosis of the superior mesenteric artery. A 22-year-old white female with a history of Takayasu arteritis is evaluated for hypertension and abdominal pain. She has a history of cold, cyanotic hands as well as pain in both lower extremities. On occasion, she also has abdominal pain. Coronal noncontrast MIP MRA shows thickening of the abdominal aortic wall and narrowing of the aortic lumen beginning at the level of the superior mesenteric artery and extending distally to the bifurcation (the narrowing is best visualized distally). She has a 60% stenosis of the proximal right renal artery (*arrow*) and an 80% to 90% stenosis of the proximal superior mesenteric artery, which is not well visualized on this image.

QUESTIONS AND ANSWERS

BOARD REVIEW QUESTIONS

1. An asymptomatic 35-year-old male presents to your office for evaluation of a heart murmur. On examination, he has an early systolic click followed by a short ejection murmur. A TTE reveals a bicuspid aortic valve with a mean transvalvular gradient of 18 mm Hg. His ascending aorta is dilated, measuring 4.2 cm in diameter. You recommend:
   A. Yearly clinical follow-up and repeat imaging every 2 years
   B. Clinical follow-up every 6 months and repeat imaging based on changes in symptoms and physical examination
   C. Yearly clinical follow-up with imaging
   D. Yearly clinical follow-up and imaging every 5 years

2. A 44-year-old female presents for a second opinion. She has a bicuspid aortic valve and mild aortic regurgitation; she takes 50 mg of long-acting metoprolol daily. She denies a history of hypertension, CAD, or cerebrovascular disease. She smokes 1 pack/day and has done so for the past 20 years. Family history is significant for a brother who died of an ascending aortic dissection at age 48. A CT scan with contrast reveals dilation of her ascending aorta, measuring 4.7 cm in diameter. You recommend:
   A. Yearly follow-up with imaging and ascending aortic aneurysm repair and aortic valve replacement when the aortic regurgitation becomes severe or the patient develops symptoms
   B. Biannual clinical follow-up with imaging and elective ascending aortic aneurysm surgical repair when the aortic diameter is >5.5 cm
   C. Proceed with elective ascending aortic aneurysm surgical repair when the aortic diameter is >5 cm
   D. Proceed with elective ascending aortic aneurysm surgical repair now

3. It is recommended that a patient (in the absence of significant risk factors such as an expansion rate >0.5 cm/year, aortic coarctation, long smoking history, or first-degree relative with ascending aortic dissection or rupture) with a bicuspid aortic valve and an ascending aortic aneurysm undergo repair of the aneurysm at an aortic diameter of:
   A. 4.0 cm
   B. 4.5 cm
   C. 5.0 cm
   D. 5.5 cm
   E. 6.0 cm

4. Surgical intervention is recommended for idiopathic ascending aortic aneurysms at an aortic diameter of:
   A. 4.5 cm
   B. 5.0 cm
   C. 5.5 cm
   D. 6.0 cm

5. The most common arrhythmia in congenital heart disease patients is:
   A. Atrial flutter
   B. Atrial tachycardia
   C. Atrial fibrillation
   D. VT

6. A 40-year-old male with a history of surgical repair of tetralogy of Fallot presents for evaluation after an episode of near-syncope. He denies any prior similar episodes. He denied feeling palpitations, chest pain, or shortness of breath with the episode. He is not limited in his activities. Echocardiogram reveals normal LV size and function. The RV is mildly dilated with mildly decreased function. A Holter monitor reveals short runs of NSVT. The next step in evaluation/management you recommend is:
   A. Exercise treadmill stress ECG with cardiac catheterization if abnormal
   B. Tilt table and pacemaker implant if abnormal
   C. Beta-blocker therapy and an implantable loop recorder if he has recurrent symptoms
   D. Detailed imaging to evaluate the pulmonic valve for stenosis or regurgitation with replacement if indicated and implantation of an ICD
   E. Detailed imaging to evaluate the pulmonic valve for stenosis or regurgitation with replacement if indicated

7. Which of the following is the most common defect associated with Ebstein anomaly?
   A. VSD
   B. ASD
   C. Bicuspid aortic valve
   D. Subaortic stenosis
   E. Mitral valve prolapse

8. Which of the following are the most common arrhythmias and/or conduction abnormalities in patients with Ebstein anomaly?
   A. First-degree AV block and AVRT (accessory pathway)
   B. Complete heart block and AVRT
   C. AVRT and atrial fibrillation
   D. Atrial flutter and VT

9. With which of the following maternal infections is PDA commonly associated?
   A. Toxoplasmosis
   B. Chicken pox
   C. Rubella
   D. Measles

10. A 50-year-old male who recently immigrated to the country presents for evaluation of episodic fevers and shortness of breath that began 1 week earlier. He denies any sick contacts or recent procedures. He complains of a dry cough, progressive shortness of breath, and intermittent sharp chest pain. His history is significant for hypertension and tobacco use. On examination, his oxygen saturation is 86% on room air, and he has diminished breath sounds in the right base. In addition, a murmur is noted at the second LICS that is present throughout the cardiac cycle. To definitively diagnose and then treat this patient, you would order:
    A. CBC, blood cultures, and chest x-ray
    B. Blood cultures and TTE
    C. Blood cultures, TEE, spiral CT of chest with contrast
    D. Blood cultures and spiral CT of chest with contrast
    E. Blood cultures and TEE

Matching

11. Subclavian artery to PA shunt

12. SVC flow redirected to the PAs (bypassing the right atrium)

13. Atrial switch operation (pulmonary venous blood "baffled" to the tricuspid valve)

14. IVC flow redirected to the PAs (bypassing the right atrium)

15. Direct anastomosis of ascending aorta to right PA

16. Arterial switch operation

    A. Mustard/Senning procedure
    B. Jantene operation
    C. Blalock-Taussig shunt
    D. Waterston shunt
    E. Hemi-Fontan procedure or Glenn shunt
    F. Fontan operation

Matching (answers may be used more than once and a numbered defect may have more than one answer)

17. D-TGA (aortic root is positioned anterior and to the right of the PA)

18. Tetralogy of Fallot

19. Tricuspid atresia

20. Pulmonary atresia and hypoplastic RV

    A. Fontan operation
    B. Arterial switch procedure
    C. Senning or Mustard procedure
    D. Closure of VSD and repair of RVOT

21. A 50-year-old patient with Fontan circulation presents for evaluation with lower extremity swelling, increasing abdominal girth, exercise intolerance, and fatigue. His current medications are digoxin and furosemide. His BP is 108/55 mm Hg, pulse 96 bpm and regular, and respiratory rate 16. On examination a grade III/VI holosystolic blowing murmur is heard at the apex. There are decreased breath sounds in the bases. Ascites is noted on abdominal examination with significant pitting edema to the knees. Which of the following tests will provide you with the most definitive information to enable a diagnosis?
    A. TTE
    B. TEE
    C. Invasive assessment in the catheterization laboratory
    D. Cardiac MRI

22. A 50-year-old diabetic male presents to your office for evaluation. He is hypertensive, but has no known CAD. He does not smoke. He is asymptomatic and states he runs 2 miles/day. Current medications include ramipril 10 mg/day and aspirin 81 mg/day. On examination, his BP is 140/80 mm Hg and pulse is 65 bpm and regular. The physical examination is unremarkable. You recommend:
    A. Add 12.5 mg of hydrochlorothiazide to his regimen
    B. Stop ramipril and begin candesartan 16 mg/day
    C. Add 25 mg of long-acting metoprolol to his regimen
    D. Stop ramipril and begin aliskiren
    E. Increase ramipril to 20 mg/day

23. A 60-year-old male with diabetes and chronic stable angina presents for routine follow-up. He denies any change in his angina pattern. His BP is 127/70 mm Hg on lisinopril/hydrochlorothiazide. He has a HbA$_{1c}$ of 6.8%. The patient's total cholesterol level is 185 mg/dL, HDL 32 mg/dL, and triglycerides 285 mg/dL. In addition to dietary changes, you recommend:
    A. No additional therapy; his calculated LDL is <100 mg/dL
    B. Having the laboratory complete a direct LDL level before recommending drug therapy
    C. Adding atorvastatin 20 mg/day to his regimen
    D. Adding fenofibrate 145 mg/day to his regimen

24. A 55-year-old male who had an anterior MI 4 years ago presents for routine follow-up. He denies any symptoms of angina or CHF. He exercises regularly. His current medications are aspirin 81 mg/day, lisinopril 10 mg/day, carvedilol 25 mg b.i.d., and atorvastatin 40 mg/day. His BP is 122/72 mm Hg, and his pulse is 60 bpm and regular. On auscultation he has a short systolic ejection murmur at the base. Lungs are clear to auscultation. His HDL is 30 mg/dL, LDL 72 mg/dL, and triglycerides 180 mg/dL. To most effectively increase his HDL, you recommend:
   A. Cholestyramine
   B. Plant sterols
   C. Fish oil
   D. Niacin
   E. Fenofibrate

25. A 66-year-old female presents to your clinic for evaluation. She has known CAD, hypertension, hyperlipidemia, gout, and diverticulosis. Her current medications include carvedilol 3.125 mg b.i.d., aspirin 81 mg/day, allopurinol 300 mg/day, and simvastatin 40 mg/day. She denies angina but complains of dyspnea on exertion and significant fatigue. On examination, she has gained 30 pounds since her last visit 1 year ago. Her BP is 110/68 mm Hg, pulse 50 bpm and regular. Heart and lung examination is unremarkable. A fasting lipid panel is completed. Total cholesterol is 300 mg/dL, LDL 180 mg/dL, and triglycerides 220 mg/dL. One year ago, her lipid levels were at goal. To further evaluate/treat the patient, you:
   A. Ensure compliance, recommend weight loss and a regular exercise program, and recheck lipids in 8–12 weeks
   B. Check serum TSH
   C. Check fasting glucose level
   D. Increase simvastatin to 80 mg/day and recommend a regular exercise program
   E. Add fenofibrate 145 mg/day and recommend a regular exercise program

26. A 58-year-old female with rheumatic heart disease presents for evaluation. She complains of dyspnea on exertion. Walking two blocks on level ground causes dyspnea. She also complains of lower extremity swelling and intermittent nausea. On examination she has a grade II/VI holosystolic murmur at her apex and a grade III/VI holosystolic murmur at the lower left sternal border. In addition, there is a grade III/VI diastolic murmur at the apex. She has decreased breath sounds in the bases and bilateral pitting edema to her knees. A TTE is completed. The mean gradient across the mitral valve is 12 mm Hg, and 2+ mitral regurgitation is noted. LV function is preserved. In addition, severe tricuspid regurgitation is noted. The tricuspid leaflets appear normal in structure, but malcoaptation is noted. This patient should:
   A. Undergo mitral valve replacement and tricuspid valve repair using an annuloplasty ring
   B. Undergo isolated mitral valve replacement; the tricuspid regurgitation will improve when the left-sided obstruction is relieved
   C. Undergo mitral balloon valvotomy and reassessment of tricuspid regurgitation after the procedure as the tricuspid regurgitation will likely improve and not require surgical intervention
   D. Undergo concomitant mitral and tricuspid valve replacement

27. The Dual Chamber and VVI Implantable Defibrillator (DAVID) trial compared dual-chamber rate responsive pacing at 70 bpm (DDDR) to ventricular backup pacing only at 40 bpm (VVI) in patients with decreased LV function. The study demonstrated that:
   A. Patients with DDDR pacing at 70 bpm had greater rates of hospitalization for heart failure compared to patients with VVI backup pacing at 40 bpm
   B. Patients with VVI backup pacing at 40 bpm had greater risk of hospitalization for heart failure or death compared to patients with DDDR pacing at 70 bpm
   C. Patients with DDDR pacing at 70 bpm had increased risk of hospitalization for heart failure and mortality compared to patients with VVI backup pacing at 40 bpm
   D. Patients with VVI backup pacing at 40 bpm had higher rates of hospitalization for heart failure but lower rates of atrial fibrillation compared to the DDDR pacing group

28. A 42-year-old Asian female presents to the hospital with dysarthria and right upper extremity weakness. While in the emergency department her symptoms begin to improve; they completely resolve during the next 12 hours. She denies any prior history of weakness but had two episodes of difficulty with word finding in the past 6 months, one after significant exertion and another after several hours in the sun. She states that she feels her memory is poor and complains of frequent, nearly daily headaches for which medications have been ineffective. MRI and MRA reveal reduced flow in the distal ICAs and the anterior and middle cerebral arteries. An extensive collateral network of vessels is also noted. Formal angiography is scheduled and you preliminarily diagnose:
    A. Agenesis of the anterior circle of Willis
    B. Moyamoya disease
    C. WAGR syndrome
    D. Multiple strokes secondary to repeated embolization

29. In the Optimal Pharmacological Therapy in Cardioverter (OPTIC)—defibrillator patients trial, which of the following medications resulted in the lowest risk of defibrillator shocks?
    A. Beta-blocker
    B. Amiodarone
    C. Sotalol
    D. Amiodarone and a beta-blocker
    E. Amiodarone and an ACE inhibitor

30. A 19-year-old male plans on playing college football. He presents to his clinician's office for evaluation before beginning practice. He is asymptomatic and denies any cardiovascular symptoms. He denies any family history of premature CAD, sudden death, hypertension, or recurrent syncope. His physical examination is normal. At this time, as his physician, you would recommend:
    A. Preparticipation exercise ECG
    B. Baseline ECG
    C. Screening CBC, urinalysis, comprehensive metabolic panel, lipid panel
    D. Preparticipation echocardiography
    E. No further testing necessary

31. A 20-year-old female has a history of rheumatic fever with carditis 5 years ago. Since beginning college 2 years ago, she has not been adhering to her prescribed antibiotic prophylaxis, and she presents to your office for follow-up because her mother insists. She is asymptomatic. She runs 4–5 miles several times per week. Her physical examination is unremarkable. Echocardiography reveals normal cardiac structures. Chamber sizes and function are also normal. You recommend:
    A. No further prophylaxis
    B. Prophylaxis with penicillin V for 1 more year
    C. Prophylaxis with benzathine penicillin for 5 more years
    D. Prophylaxis with benzathine penicillin until age 40
    E. Prophylaxis with penicillin V for 10 more years

32. A 67-year-old female presents to her cardiologist for follow-up. She states that her weight has been stable and denies orthopnea. She continues to have significant dyspnea on exertion, complaining of dyspnea after walking one flight of stairs or two to three blocks. She also complains of a persistent dry cough. She states it developed approximately 4 months ago around the time of her last visit. She is currently taking ramipril, metoprolol, aspirin, furosemide, and digoxin. The cardiologist stops ramipril and decides to initiate an ARB that has been proven to reduce cardiovascular death in heart failure. The cardiologist chooses:
    A. Irbesartan
    B. Candesartan
    C. Telmisartan
    D. Losartan

33. A 48-year-old female presents to the emergency department with complaints of a painful and swollen right calf. Venous Doppler studies confirm the diagnosis of a DVT of the right popliteal vein extending into the superficial femoral vein. The patient denies any recent travel or surgery in the past 6 months. She does not smoke. She has not been to a physician or hospital in the past 12 years. There is no family history of thromboembolic disease. The patient is placed on warfarin. Enoxaparin is also administered until she is therapeutic on warfarin. As her physician, you recommend:
    A. CT of the chest, abdomen, and pelvis to screen for occult malignancy
    B. CT of the chest and tumor marker levels to screen for malignancy
    C. Complete history and physical examination, routine laboratory tests, and chest x-ray
    D. Complete history and physical examination, routine laboratory tests, chest x-ray, Pap smear, and breast mammography

34. A 36-year-old male complains of chest pain that has been present for 3 days. He describes it as sharp and worse when he lies down. He also relates he has had a low-grade fever and significant fatigue in the past 3 days. An ECG reveals diffuse concave ST-segment elevation, sparing lead aV_R. In addition, PR depression is noted in the inferior leads. An echocardiogram reveals a small pericardial effusion. A CBC, general chemistries, and chest x-ray are unremarkable. He denies smoking or alcohol use, and has not traveled recently. He denies any other medical problems and does not take any medications. He has never had any similar symptoms. You recommend:
    A. Aspirin or NSAID therapy
    B. Aspirin or NSAID therapy and systemic steroids
    C. Colchicine
    D. Steroids
    E. Aspirin or NSAID therapy plus colchicine

35. Which of the following is the most common primary cardiac tumor?
   A. Sarcoma
   B. Lipoma
   C. Papillary fibroelastoma
   D. Myxoma

36. Which of the following is the most common malignant primary cardiac tumor?
   A. Angiosarcoma
   B. Cardiac lymphoma
   C. Rhabdomyosarcoma
   D. Fibrosarcoma
   E. Osteosarcoma

37. The omega-3 fatty acids EPA and DHA, found in fatty fish or supplements, have been shown to:
   A. Lower LDL levels
   B. Lower triglyceride levels
   C. Lower LDL and triglyceride levels
   D. Lower triglyceride levels and raise LDL levels
   E. Lower LDL levels and raise HDL levels

38. In the Acute Catheterization and Urgent Intervention Triage Strategy (ACUITY) trial, patients treated with bivalirudin compared to UFH/enoxaparin and a glycoprotein IIb/IIIa inhibitor had:
   A. A decrease in ischemic end points and no difference in major bleeding
   B. No difference in ischemic end points and a decrease in major bleeding
   C. No difference in ischemic end points or major bleeding
   D. An increase in ischemic end points and no difference in major bleeding
   E. No difference in ischemic end points and an increase in major bleeding

39. A 56-year-old female with diabetes presents for a second opinion. She underwent cardiac catheterization after an NSTEMI. This revealed an 80% proximal LAD lesion and a 90% mid-RCA lesion. LV function is preserved by left ventriculography. Her last HbA_{1c} was 7.5%. Her LDL is 99 mg/dL. She currently takes aspirin, metoprolol, ramipril, atorvastatin, and levamir insulin. According to the 10-year results of the Bypass Angioplasty Revascularization Investigation (BARI) trial, you recommend:
   A. She undergo two-vessel drug-eluting stent placement or CABG, which both provide the same results
   B. She undergo two-vessel drug-eluting stent placement
   C. She undergo CABG
   D. She undergo neither CABG nor stent placement; her medical therapy should be further optimized and she should undergo an ischemia evaluation before any procedure is performed

40. A 75-year-old female is admitted to the hospital with shortness of breath and edema. She has dilated cardiomyopathy with an ejection fraction of 25%. This is her fourth hospitalization in 6 months. She has been dyspneic at rest for the past several months, but it significantly worsened over the past 48 hours. She can no longer cook her own meals or do any housework because of fatigue and shortness of breath. She follows a low-sodium diet and adheres to her medical regimen. She had an ICD placed 5 years ago. She has experienced two appropriate ICD discharges in the past 6 months. Current medications include metoprolol succinate 100 mg/day, ramipril 10 mg b.i.d., digoxin 0.125 mg/day, and furosemide 80 mg b.i.d. On examination, her BP is 104/62 mm Hg, pulse 72 bpm, and respiratory rate 20. Cardiovascular examination reveals a diffuse PMI, normal heart sounds, and a grade III/VI holosystolic murmur at the apex. Rales are heard in the lower one third of her lung fields. She has 2+ pitting edema at her ankles. Laboratory data reveals a Hb of 11.4 g/dL, Na 132 mmol/L, K 4 mmol/L, BUN 40 mg/dL, Cr 2 mg/dL, and CHF peptide of 1600 pg/mL. Your next action is to:
   A. Arrange intermittent home dobutamine infusions
   B. Place a Swan-Ganz catheter to better adjust her diuretic dose
   C. Discuss with the patient the option of turning off her defibrillator
   D. Begin spironolactone 12.5 mg/day
   E. Transfer the patient to a nursing home for end-of-life care

41. A 65-year-old African American female presents to clinic for follow-up. She has ischemic cardiomyopathy with an ejection fraction of 35%. She had a three-vessel CABG 5 years ago. She has class III symptoms, describing difficulty in performing her daily activities. She recently was admitted for an exacerbation of heart failure. She underwent an adenosine myocardial perfusion scan that revealed a small apical infarct but no ischemia. An echocardiogram revealed akinesis of her apex and severe mitral regurgitation. Current medications include metoprolol succinate, digoxin, furosemide, lisinopril, and aspirin. On examination, BP is 132/70 mm Hg, heart rate 72 bpm, respiratory rate 16, weight 200 pounds, and BMI 32. Chest is clear to auscultation, and there is a grade III/VI holosystolic murmur at her apex. Mild peripheral edema is noted. Your next step in management is:
   A. Place a Holter monitor to evaluate for significant arrhythmia contributing to her heart failure
   B. Refer the patient for mitral valve annuloplasty
   C. Add hydralazine and isosorbide to her medical regimen
   D. Add candesartan to her medical regimen
   E. Switch the metoprolol to carvedilol

42. You are asked to consult on a 48-year-old male with dilated cardiomyopathy. He has functional class III symptoms. A cardiac catheterization 5 years ago revealed mild irregularities of his coronary arteries. ECG reveals sinus rhythm, LAD, and an IVCD measuring 118 msec. Echocardiogram reveals a moderately dilated LV, and dysynchronous contraction of the septum and posterior wall is noted. Ejection fraction is estimated at 30%. He has not been hospitalized in over one year. Current medications include carvedilol, candesartan, enalapril, and furosemide. Physical examination finds a BP of 130/80 mm Hg, pulse 72 bpm and regular, and respiratory rate of 16. Heart sounds are distant and no murmur is auscultated. Lung sounds are normal and his jugular venous pulse is not elevated. Your next step in management of this patient would be:
    A. Add spironolactone to his regimen
    B. Place a biventricular pacemaker/ICD
    C. Add digoxin to his regimen
    D. Titrate up his carvedilol
    E. Increase his furosemide dose

43. Which of the following patients has an absolute indication for cardiac transplant?
    A. A 40-year-old female with an ejection fraction of 15% and class III–IV symptoms of CHF
    B. A 60-year-old male with ischemic cardiomyopathy, ejection fraction of 30%, and persistent anginal symptoms on maximal medical therapy that limits his daily activity not amenable to CABG or PCI
    C. A 55-year-old male with dilated cardiomyopathy, ejection fraction of 25%, and recurrent episodes of fluid retention despite compliance with prescribed diet and medical regimen
    D. A 64-year-old female with cardiomyopathy, ejection fraction of 25%, and peak VO_2 of 12 mL/kg/min

44. Which of the following is an effect of antiarrhythmic drugs that can lead to torsades de pointes?
    A. Delayed afterdepolarizations
    B. Hyperkalemia
    C. Hypermagnesemia
    D. Early afterdepolarizations

45. A 52-year-old male presents with atrial fibrillation of 16 hours' duration. He has no known heart disease. His examination is unremarkable except for an irregular rhythm at a rate of 122 bpm. A decision is made to try to terminate his episode of atrial fibrillation with I.V. antiarrhythmic medication. Which of the following medications is approved for this indication?
    A. Amiodarone
    B. Disopyramide
    C. Dofetilide
    D. Ibutilide
    E. Propafenone

46. A 75-year-old male presents to the hospital after experiencing ICD shocks. He has a history of ischemic cardiomyopathy. His ejection fraction is 35%. Six months ago he had two ICD shocks 2 weeks apart. He is currently on carvedilol 25 mg b.i.d., furosemide 40 mg b.i.d., KCl 20 mEq b.i.d., aspirin 81 mg/day, quinapril 10 mg b.i.d., and atorvastatin 40 mg/day. Examination reveals an elderly male in no acute distress. He is alert and oriented. Heart is regular with a grade III/VI holosystolic murmur at the apex. Lungs are clear to auscultation, and there is trace peripheral edema. His device is interrogated, and all of the ICD shocks are found to be appropriate. The current episode of VT terminated after three shocks. When his device was placed 1 year ago, he underwent defibrillation threshold testing, and his device was set at maximum output for each shock delivered. As you discuss further treatment options with him, you recommend the initiation of an antiarrhythmic medication. In this situation, you choose to initiate:
    A. Sotalol
    B. Amiodarone
    C. Procainamide
    D. Propafenone

47. A 28-year-old asymptomatic male is referred to you for evaluation. His PCP did an ECG, which revealed pre-excitation. The patient relates that he occasionally feels a flutter in his chest. One year ago he experienced a 20-minute episode of palpitations that spontaneously resolved. His PCP told him he could die suddenly if he did not undergo an ablation. He tells you that he does not want an invasive procedure unless he is at high risk of dying. You recommend:
    A. Placing a 48-hour Holter monitor to detect asymptomatic arrhythmias
    B. Performing exercise ECG
    C. Performing an EP study
    D. No further testing; reassurance only

48. Which of the following diseases characterized by syncope, VT, and sudden death results from a mutation in the cardiac sodium channel gene (*SCN5A*) leading to a loss of function or reduction in the sodium current?
    A. Long QT syndrome 1
    B. Long QT syndrome 2
    C. Long QT syndrome 3
    D. Brugada syndrome

49. Match the syndrome with the situation in which sudden death is likely to occur. Answers may be used more than once.
    1. Long QT syndrome 1
    2. Long QT syndrome 2
    3. Long QT syndrome 3
    4. Brugada syndrome
    A. Loud noise/emotional stimuli
    B. Exercise, especially swimming
    C. Sleep/rest

50. In the Surgical Treatment for Ischemic Heart Failure (STICH) trial, CABG alone was compared to CABG plus surgical ventricular reconstruction. The results were:
    A. Increased mortality and decreased exercise tolerance
    B. Decreased mortality and increased exercise tolerance
    C. No difference in either mortality or exercise tolerance
    D. Increased mortality but no difference in exercise tolerance
    E. No difference in mortality and increased exercise tolerance

51. Which of the following is the most common cause of syncope in the middle-aged?
    A. Ventricular arrhythmias
    B. Cardiac medications
    C. Neurocardiogenic syncope
    D. Obstruction to cardiac output

52. Which of the following steps in the evaluation of syncope has the greatest diagnostic yield?
    A. History and physical examination
    B. Holter monitor
    C. ECG
    D. Echocardiogram

53. A 56-year-old male is brought by ambulance to the emergency department after an episode of transient loss of consciousness. He was walking down the hall talking to a co-worker when he collapsed. The co-worker states that he stopped talking and then collapsed. He struck his head when he fell and has a large ecchymosis over his right temple. The co-worker describes rhythmic jerking of the patient's arms and legs for approximately 60 seconds after his collapse. The patient denies any prodromal symptoms such as diaphoresis, nausea, or palpitations. The patient has been diabetic for approximately 3 years. He smokes 1 pack of cigarettes per day. Examination reveals a pulse of 82 bpm, BP of 145/90 mm Hg, and a grade II/VI early peaking systolic ejection murmur at the base. ECG reveals normal sinus rhythm with several PVCs. An echocardiogram is completed, which reveals normal-sized cardiac chambers, mild concentric LVH, estimated ejection fraction of 60%, and aortic sclerosis. You are called to the emergency department in consultation. You recommend:
    A. Placement of a Holter monitor
    B. No further evaluation necessary
    C. Admission with telemetry and EEG
    D. Exercise ECG
    E. Carotid Doppler studies

54. All of the following statements regarding adult patients presenting with sudden onset of severe LV failure within 2 weeks of a viral illness and who have typical lymphocytic myocarditis on EMB are true EXCEPT:
    A. These patients have a poor prognosis.
    B. These patients are often in cardiogenic shock.
    C. The LV is often thick but not dilated.
    D. Intravenous inotropes or mechanical assistance is often required for circulatory support.

55. A 44-year-old white male presents to the hospital with dyspnea. He states he first started to develop shortness of breath 1 month ago during his daily 2-mile walks. Three weeks ago he saw his physician, who started him on furosemide and an ACE inhibitor for cardiomegaly on chest x-ray and mild pulmonary edema. One week later he was initiated on carvedilol. However, his symptoms have worsened; now he is short of breath with his daily activities. He has orthopnea and paroxysmal nocturnal dyspnea. Past medical history is significant for untreated rheumatoid arthritis and tobacco use. Physical examination reveals a heart rate of 110 bpm and BP of 100/60 mm Hg. His PMI is difficult to palpate. His internal jugular veins are moderately distended, heart is regular, and an S_3 is auscultated. A grade II/VI holosystolic murmur is heard at the apex. 2+ pitting edema is noted in his lower extremities. ECG reveals sinus rhythm and nonspecific ST-segment and T-wave changes. On telemetry he has multiple runs of NSVT. Echocardiogram reveals a moderately dilated LV with an ejection fraction of 20%. Diagnostic coronary angiography reveals normal coronary arteries. An EMB is performed. The EMB is most likely to demonstrate:
    A. Patchy myocyte necrosis and inflammation with a lymphocytic infiltrate
    B. Diffuse inflammation with a predominant number of eosinophils
    C. Widespread necrosis, lymphocytes, eosinophils, and multinucleated giant cells
    D. Multinucleated giant cells, noncaseating granulomas, and sparse necrosis

56. With the diagnosis established, you then immediately elect to:
    A. Add digoxin and spironolactone to his therapy
    B. Begin multidrug immunosuppressive therapy
    C. Begin I.V. amiodarone
    D. Begin corticosteroids

57. Many age-related changes predispose the elderly to syncope. All of the following are changes related to aging EXCEPT:
    A. Loss of peripheral autonomic tone
    B. Reduction in thirst
    C. An increase in the baroreceptor response
    D. Reduction in ability to preserve Na and water

58. A 46-year-old female presents for evaluation after an episode of syncope. She was running around the track at the gym when she collapsed. Witnesses report that she aroused quickly after collapsing. She bruised her forehead and left shoulder. She denies any premonitory symptoms, palpitations, or chest pain. She has had no prior similar events. She just began exercising regularly 2 months ago. She has hypertension and hypothyroidism. She takes hydrochlorothiazide and levothyroxine daily. Her ECG shows sinus rhythm without other abnormalities. Her physical examination shows a heart rate of 78 bpm and BP of 138/85 mm Hg, otherwise unremarkable. An echocardiogram and adenosine myocardial perfusion scan are normal. As the consulting cardiologist, you elect to:
    A. Send her home with an event monitor
    B. Place an implantable loop recorder
    C. Perform an EP study
    D. No further testing; reevaluate in 1 month
    E. Change her hydrochlorothiazide to amlodipine

59. A patient with known CAD and prior NSTEMI has an episode of unexplained syncope. Cardiac stress testing does not reveal any ischemia. The patient should then undergo an EP study for further evaluation. **True or false?**

60. A 39-year-old female presents to a rural hospital 2 hours after the acute onset of severe chest pressure radiating to her left arm. She has no significant past medical history. She is 6 weeks postpartum and is breast-feeding her infant. On examination, her heart is regular with an S_3 gallop. She has crackles in her bases bilaterally. No peripheral edema is noted. An ECG shows ST-segment elevation in the anterior leads. The nearest catheterization laboratory is 45 minutes away. You proceed to:
    A. Transfer the patient for immediate coronary angiography and PCI
    B. Administer thrombolytic therapy and then transfer to the tertiary hospital for rescue PCI if needed
    C. Administer nitroglycerin intravenously; give oral aspirin and metoprolol and repeat the ECG and assessment in 30 minutes to see if the ST-segment elevation resolves
    D. Begin heparin and nitroglycerin intravenously and transfer to the tertiary hospital for emergent angiography

61. A 60-year-old female presents to the emergency department with severe sudden-onset chest pain 3 hours earlier. She states the pain began after an argument with her sister on the telephone. She has a history of hypertension and takes ramipril to treat it. She denies diabetes, hyperlipidemia or tobacco use. Her father had an MI at age 57. In the emergency department, she is given oxygen, aspirin, nitroglycerin, and heparin; 30 minutes later, her pain is rated a 2 out of 10 in severity. You come to evaluate her and find on examination that her pulse is 96 bpm and regular, BP 100/62 mm Hg, oxygen saturation 94% on 2 L of oxygen. Heart is regular with a normal S_1 and S_2. There is a grade III/VI midpeaking systolic ejection murmur at her left midsternal border and a grade II/VI holosystolic blowing murmur at her apex radiating to her back. She has bilateral crackles over her lower lung fields, but no peripheral edema. Her ECG reveals sinus rhythm with deep symmetric precordial T-wave inversions with prolongation of the QT interval. The most likely etiologies of her murmurs are:
    A. Mild aortic stenosis and mitral valve prolapsed
    B. Mild aortic stenosis and ischemic mitral regurgitation
    C. Dynamic outflow tract obstruction and mitral regurgitation
    D. Dynamic outflow tract obstruction and ischemic mitral regurgitation

62. After evaluating the patient in the emergency department, you immediately elect to:
    A. Proceed to emergent coronary angiography and PCI
    B. Obtain a stat echocardiogram
    C. Administer I.V. furosemide
    D. Administer intravenous beta-blocker and a normal saline bolus

63. The most common ECG change in patients with intracranial bleeding or ischemic stroke is:
    A. QT-interval prolongation
    B. ST-segment depression
    C. Development of U waves
    D. T-wave inversions

64. A 60-year-old male with unstable angina underwent cardiac catheterization, which revealed severe three-vessel CAD. His past history is significant for diabetes, hypertension, hyperlipidemia, asthma, and gout. His current medications include metformin, glyburide, lisinopril, amlodipine, aspirin, albuterol, salmeterol, and allopurinol. On examination, pulse is 85 bpm and regular, BP is 158/90 mm Hg, and respiratory rate is 16. There is a grade II/VI holosystolic murmur at his apex. Lungs are clear without wheezing or crackles. He has minimal lower-extremity swelling. ECG displays sinus rhythm, with PACs, LAE, and voltage for LVH. TTE revealed he had moderate concentric LVH, ejection fraction of 45%, moderate LAE, and mild to moderate mitral regurgitation. The patient is referred for CABG. In an attempt to most effectively decrease postoperative complications, you recommend:
    A. The addition of low-dose beta-blocker that is continued lifelong
    B. The addition of a statin that is continued lifelong
    C. A mitral valve annuloplasty ring to be placed at the time of CABG
    D. The addition of amiodarone now and postoperatively
    E. An insulin drip postoperatively to control blood glucose

65. All of the following pharmacologic interventions have some data demonstrating efficacy in decreasing the incidence of atrial fibrillation EXCEPT:
    A. Atorvastatin
    B. Omega-3 polyunsaturated fatty acids
    C. Magnesium
    D. Digoxin
    E. Hydrocortisone

66. A 45-year-old male presents for evaluation after two episodes of syncope, one of which occurred after eating at a restaurant as he stood to leave and the other while he was stacking boxes on a shelf at work. There is no family history of sudden cardiac death or premature CAD. He takes no medications. His baseline ECG displays sinus rhythm with an RSR′ in V_1. A repeat ECG is obtained with the V_1 lead at the second ICS; there was no significant change. A maximal Bruce protocol exercise stress test is without evidence of ischemia. He exercised for 10 minutes. An echocardiogram reveals a structurally normal heart and normal LV and RV function. At a follow-up visit, you obtain an ECG. He states that he just finished eating a very large meal. The ECG displays a type 1 ECG pattern of Brugada syndrome. You recommend:
    A. Placement of an ICD
    B. Placement of an implantable loop recorder
    C. 48-hour Holter monitoring
    D. No further testing; initiation of medical therapy
    E. EP study with placement of ICD or pacemaker if indicated

67. The patient declines any further testing or procedures. He states that he fully understands the risk of not undergoing any further evaluation and that he is willing to take a medication to treat his condition if it may be helpful. Therefore, you prescribe:
    A. Amiodarone
    B. Metoprolol
    C. Quinidine
    D. Isoproterenol
    E. Dofetilide

68. Serum levels of B-type natriuretic peptide are lower in patients with obesity and therefore B-type natriuretic peptide is not a reliable marker for heart failure in this patient population. **True or false?**

69. According to published studies, which of the following statements about bariatric surgery is true?
    A. It results in long-term weight loss of up to 40%.
    B. It results in an improvement in hypertension in >50% of patients.
    C. It results in an improvement in lipid status in >50% of patients.
    D. It results in a resolution or improvement of diabetes in >50% of patients.
    E. All of the above.

70. What is the threshold value of indexed prosthetic valve EOA generally used to define severe PPM in the aortic position?
    A. $<1 \text{ cm}^2/\text{m}^2$
    B. $<0.85 \text{ cm}^2/\text{m}^2$
    C. $<0.65 \text{ cm}^2/\text{m}^2$
    D. $<0.5 \text{ cm}^2/\text{m}^2$

71. A 72-year-old obese male with hypertension, hyperlipidemia, and a history of tobacco use underwent bare metal stent placement to his proximal LAD 6 weeks ago. He had been experiencing chest discomfort, and results of an exercise stress test were abnormal. He denies any recurrence of his symptoms. His medications include metoprolol 25 mg b.i.d., aspirin 325 mg/day, clopidogrel 75 mg/day, atorvastatin 40 mg/day, and furosemide 40 mg/day. The patient returned to the hospital yesterday evening with abdominal discomfort and nausea. Abdominal imaging has identified cholelithiasis with moderate edema and thickening of the gallbladder wall. His temperature is 100.4°F (38°C), pulse 90 bpm and regular, and BP 142/85 mm Hg. His ECG is unchanged from his prior tracing 1 month ago. The general surgeon has recommended cholecystectomy and wants to discontinue the patient's aspirin and clopidogrel. He thinks he may need to do a laparotomy instead of a laparoscopic procedure. You are called to consult before the planned surgery. You recommend:

    A. Proceed with surgery but recommend that the patient remain on aspirin and clopidogrel at current doses.
    B. Stop clopidogrel and continue aspirin at 81 mg/day in the perioperative period. Proceed with surgery and restart clopidogrel as soon as possible after the procedure.
    C. Stop clopidogrel and continue aspirin at 81 mg/day. Begin I.V. heparin at therapeutic doses and discontinue it 4 hours before surgery. Restart heparin postoperatively as soon as possible. Restart clopidogrel and discontinue heparin when the surgeon is comfortable.
    D. Stop clopidogrel. Continue aspirin at 81 mg/day. Proceed with surgery and begin glycoprotein IIb/IIIa inhibitor immediately postoperatively and continue for 24 hours. Do not restart clopidogrel but continue lifelong aspirin.
    E. Discontinue aspirin and clopidogrel, and restart both as soon as possible after surgery.

72. Which of the following is a class I indication for perioperative management of a patient undergoing noncardiac surgery?

    A. Beta-blockers are recommended for patients undergoing vascular surgery in whom preoperative assessment identifies CAD.
    B. Beta-blockers are recommended for patients in whom preoperative assessment for vascular surgery identifies high cardiac risk, as defined by the presence of more than one clinical risk factor.
    C. For patients undergoing noncardiac surgery who are currently taking statins, statins should be continued.
    D. Intraoperative nitroglycerin should be used prophylacticly to prevent myocardial ischemia in high-risk patients undergoing noncardiac surgery.

73. A 69-year-old white male with a history of hypertension and diabetes mellitus experienced acute onset of chest pain and shortness of breath while mowing his lawn. After 90 minutes of discomfort, he called emergency services. On paramedic's arrival, a 12-lead ECG was obtained and revealed an anterior STEMI. The patient's pulse is 120 bpm, BP is 80/62 mm Hg, and respiratory rate is 24. His oxygen saturation is 88% on room air. The patient is given 162 mg of chewable aspirin. What is the next best step in management?

    A. Deliver fibrinolytic therapy en route to the hospital.
    B. Transfer to a hospital capable of rapid revascularization.
    C. Initate heparin and a glycoprotein IIb/IIIa inhibitor.
    D. Deliver fibrinolytic therapy on arrival at the hospital.

74. Which of the following statements concerning patients who are candidates for PCI or fibrinolysis is true?

    A. In patients selected for PCI, door to balloon time should be less than 120 minutes.
    B. In patients selected for fibrinolysis, door to needle time should be less than 30 minutes.
    C. In patients selected for fibrinolysis, door to needle time should be less than 60 minutes.
    D. In patients selected for PCI, door to balloon time should be less than 60 minutes.

75. Which of the following does not represent a class I recommendation in the treatment and evaluation of a patient with an STEMI?

    A. In patients with inferior STEMI, right-sided ECG leads should be obtained to screen for ST-segment elevation suggestive of RV infarct.
    B. A brief, focused and limited neurologic examination to look for evidence of prior stroke or cognitive deficits should be performed on STEMI patients before administration of fibrinolytic therapy.
    C. It is reasonable to administer I.V. beta-blockers promptly to STEMI patients without contraindications, especially if a tachyarrhythmia or hypertension is present.
    D. For patients with ST-segment elevation on 12-lead ECG and symptoms of STEMI, reperfusion therapy should be initiated as soon as possible and is not contigent on a bedside biomarker assay.

76. Regarding fibrinolysis versus an invasive strategy in patients with STEMI, if the time of onset of symptoms is <3 hours and there is no delay to an invasive strategy, either approach is acceptable. **True or false?**

77. Which of the following is an absolute contraindication to fibrinolytic therapy for STEMI?
    A. Pregnancy
    B. Major surgery (<3 weeks)
    C. Known structural cerebrovascular lesion (e.g., AVM)
    D. Active peptic ulcer
    E. Recent (within 2–4 weeks) internal bleeding

78. 24 hours after successful fibrinolysis of an inferior STEMI, a 62-year-old male has multiple sustained episodes of VT. By echocardiogram, his ejection fraction is estimated at 40%. What is the next best step?
    A. Implantation of an ICD before discharge
    B. Proceed to the catheterization laboratory for coronary angiography and possible coronary intervention
    C. Initiation of long-term amiodarone therapy
    D. Continuing current treatment; the VT represents reperfusion arrhythmia

79. A 47-year-old white female presented to the hospital within 3 hours of chest pain. ECG revealed anterior STEMI, and the patient received fibrinolytic therapy. After 90 minutes postinfusion of tenecteplase, the patient's ECG demonstrates 60% improvement of the initial ST-segment elevation and she is hemodynamically stable. However, she continues to have chest pain rated a 7 out of 10 in severity. What is the next best step in management?
    A. Administer a loading dose of clopidogrel 300 mg and continue clopidogrel 75 mg/day for 1 year.
    B. Improvement in ST-segment elevation and hemodynamic stability indicate successful reperfusion. Administer I.V. nitroglycerin and morphine for pain relief.
    C. Send the patient for immediate angiography and PCI.
    D. Continue close observation, and repeat ECG in 30 minutes.

80. A 57-year-old white male with a history of hypertension and diabetes presents to the emergency department with 6 hours of crushing chest pain. ECG demonstrates an anterolateral STEMI. Pulse is 92 bpm and BP is 100/60 mm Hg. He is taken urgently to the catheterization laboratory. Which of the following medications would you *not* give as initial therapy in the emergency department before transfer to the catheterization laboratory?
    A. Clopidogrel 600 mg oral loading dose
    B. Heparin 60 U/kg I.V. bolus followed by heparin infusion
    C. One dose of metoprolol 5 mg I.V.
    D. Aspirin 325 mg chewed

81. A 56-year-old African American male presented to the hospital 8 hours after developing chest pain. ECG revealed an anterior STEMI, and the patient went emergently to the cardiac catheterization laboratory. He received a drug-eluting stent to his subtotally occluded mid-LAD lesion. Echocardiogram on hospital day 2 reveals an akinetic anterior segment with an ejection fraction of 35%. Before discharge, which of the following would be appropriate?
    A. ICD implantation
    B. Institution of warfarin therapy and continuation for the next 3 months
    C. Daily NSAID therapy
    D. EP study followed by ICD placement if appropriate

82. A 72-year-old female develops recurrent chest pain 12 days after hospitalization for STEMI. Her ECG is unchanged compared to an ECG obtained before her discharge. Echocardiogram reveals a moderate pericardial effusion. On examination, BP is 118/70 mm Hg, pulsus paradoxus is 10 mm Hg, pulse 76 bpm and regular, and respiratory rate 18. A pericardial friction rub is noted. Lungs are clear to auscultation and there is no peripheral edema. Which of the following is the next best step in her management?
    A. Pericardiocentesis
    B. Discontinue aspirin and clopidogrel
    C. Aspirin 650 mg orally every 4–6 hours
    D. Ibuprofen 600 mg orally t.i.d.
    E. Prednisone 40 mg orally for 3 days and then a 2-week taper

83. A 69-year-old female develops sustained monomorphic VT 2 days after an acute inferior STEMI for which she had received fibrinolytic therapy. Her BP is 120/78 mm Hg. She is alert and denies chest pain. Her lungs are clear to auscultation, and she has no peripheral edema. Of the choices below, which treatment is indicated initially?
    A. Unsynchronized biphasic shock of 200 J repeated two additional times, if necessary
    B. Procainamide bolus and infusion
    C. Synchronized cardioversion starting at monophasic energies of 50 J
    D. Emergent catheterization

84. A 70-year-old male presented to the hospital within 2 hours of the onset of chest pain. ECG reveals ST-segment elevation in the anterior leads. BP is 160/70 mm Hg, heart rate 88 bpm, and respiratory rate 20. On examination, his heart is regular with a grade II/VI systolic ejection murmur and an S_4 gallop. Lungs are clear to auscultation, and there is no peripheral edema. The patient has no neurologic deficits. After excluding contraindications, the emergency department physician administers alteplase. The patient is then transferred to a facility capable of performing PCI. Three hours after fibrinolytic therapy, the patient becomes drowsy and is difficult to arouse. The most appropriate next step in management is:
    A. Obtain STAT CT scan of brain
    B. Obtain emergent neurosurgery consultation
    C. Intubate and hyperventilate the patient
    D. Stop I.V. heparin and aspirin
    E. Administer emergently FFP and protamine

85. Which of the following therapies is reasonable in the setting of a STEMI and subsequent hospital care of the patient?
    A. Beyond the first 48 hours after STEMI, topical nitrates for persistent CHF
    B. I.V. enalapril during the first 24 hours of STEMI for treatment of hypertension
    C. Routine use of antiarrhythmic drugs to suppress NSVT
    D. Vitamin E or vitamin C supplementation prescribed at discharge

86. A 65-year-old diabetic and hypertensive female presents to a rural emergency department after 6 hours of chest discomfort. Her home medications include lisinopril, hydrochlorothiazide, metoprolol, aspirin, glipizide, metformin, and atorvastatin. Initial ECG reveals ST-segment elevation in the inferior leads. Right-sided ECG demonstrates ST elevation in lead V4R. Initial vital signs show a BP of 95/60 mm Hg, pulse of 95 bpm and regular, and respiratory rate of 20. Her periphery is cool, and she states that she feels dizzy. She is given aspirin, alteplase, and UFH. Sixty minutes after thrombolysis her chest pain is rated a 1 out of 10 in severity. Her repeat ECG shows >50% decrease in the ST-segment elevation. All of her antihypertensive medications are held, and she is given a 1-L bolus of normal saline solution and then an infusion of 150 mL/hour of fluid. She is transferred to a tertiary care facility and 5 hours later undergoes coronary angiography, which reveals a 90% proximal RCA lesion, 80% mid-LAD lesion, and an 80% lesion in the first obtuse marginal branch of the LCX. In the catheterization laboratory, her BP is stable at 110/72 mm Hg, and heart rate is 80 bpm. An ECG is completed and the patient's left ventricular ejection fraction is estimated at 35%. The RV is noted to be moderately dilated with mildly decreased systolic function. The next most appropriate step in management is:
    A. PCI of the infarct-related artery; re-evaluation of her ejection fraction and stress testing in 4–6 weeks
    B. PCI of the RCA and a right heart catheterization to obtain a PCWP to help tailor further management
    C. IABP inserted after PCI of the infarct-related artery to increase coronary perfusion and prevent ischemia
    D. Recommend CABG surgery before discharge
    E. Recommend patient return for elective CABG surgery 1 month after discharge

87. A 68-year-old male with a history of chronic stable angina presents with chest discomfort and mild dyspnea on exertion. He develops discomfort after walking 4–5 blocks. He denies any discomfort at rest or pain with his usual daily activities. His previous ECGs have demonstrated sinus rhythm with a LBBB, and his current tracing is similar but LAD is now present. You recommend:
    A. Coronary angiography
    B. Exercise ECG
    C. Exercise stress echocardiogram
    D. Adenosine myocardial perfusion scan
    E. Dobutamine stress echocardiogram

88. A 76-year-old white female with a history of hypertension, hypothyroidism, and a GI bleed secondary to peptic ulcer disease is admitted with an NSTEMI. Her ECG demonstrates sinus tachycardia with 1 mm of ST-segment depression in the anterior lateral leads. Vital signs include BP of 115/82 mm Hg, heart rate of 112 bpm, and respiratory rate of 16. On examination, she is alert, oriented, and slightly anxious. Heart is regular with a grade II/VI systolic ejection murmur. Lungs are clear to auscultation, and there is no peripheral edema. While in the emergency department medical therapy is initiated. All of the following medications would be appropriate in the initial management of this patient EXCEPT:
    A. Heparin 60 U/kg bolus I.V. followed by 12 U/kg infusion
    B. Enoxaparin 1 mg/kg subcutaneously
    C. Metoprolol 25 mg orally
    D. Clopidogrel 300 mg oral loading dose

89. The above-mentioned patient is selected to receive a conservative strategy. Which of the following anticoagulants would not be indicated?
    A. UFH
    B. Enoxaparin
    C. Fondaparinux
    D. Bivalirudin

90. The above-mentioned patient is placed on fondaparinux and other appropriate medical therapy. When should fondaparinux be discontinued?
    A. After 24 hours
    B. After 48 hours
    C. At hospital discharge regardless of length of stay
    D. At hospital discharge or day 4, whichever is sooner
    E. At hospital discharge or day 8, whichever is sooner

91. A 77-year-old male with a history of diabetes mellitus, atrial fibrillation, and hypertension was hospitalized for an NSTEMI. He underwent angiography and received a drug-eluting stent to the culprit vessel. He has no prior history of anemia or GI bleeding. Which of the following long-term anticoagulant therapy choices would be most appropriate?
    A. Aspirin 75–162 mg/day indefinitely, clopidogrel 75 mg/day for at least 1 month and ideally up to 1 year, warfarin with a goal INR of 2–2.5
    B. Aspirin 162–325 mg/day for at least 1 month, then 75–162 mg/day indefinitely, clopidogrel 75 mg/day for at least 1 month and ideally up to 1 year, warfarin with a goal INR of 2–3
    C. Aspirin 162–325 mg/day for at least 3–6 month, then 75–162 mg/day indefinitely, clopidogrel 75 mg/day for at least 1 year, warfarin with a goal INR of 2–3
    D. Aspirin 162–325 mg/day for at least 3–6 month, then 75–162 mg/day indefinitely, clopidogrel 75 mg/day for at least 1 year, warfarin with a goal INR of 2–2.5

92. A 68-year-old male presents with an NSTEMI, and coronary angiography with possible PCI is planned. All of the following anticoagulant strategies would be appropriate EXCEPT:
    A. Bivalirudin 0.1 mg/kg I.V. bolus, then 0.25 mg/kg/hr infusion
    B. Fondaparinux 2.5 mg subcutaneously qd + UFH 60 U/kg I.V. bolus, then 12 U/kg infusion
    C. Fondaparinux 2.5 mg subcutaneously
    D. Enoxaparin 30 mg I.V. bolus followed by 1 mg/kg subcutaneously

93. All of the following statements describe characteristics of variant (Prinzmetal) angina EXCEPT:
    A. Anginal discomfort usually occurs at rest.
    B. Prolonged vasospasm may result in AV block.
    C. Anginal discomfort is more common in the early mornings.
    D. The key to diagnosis is documentation of coronary vasospasm in the cardiac catheterization laboratory.
    E. Prolonged vasospasm can result in sudden death.

94. A 35-year-old female presents with exertional dyspnea after walking 3–4 blocks. She denies any prior significant past medical history. She does not take any medications. Examination reveals an obese white female, with a BMI of 36 kg/m^2, BP of 130/85 mm Hg, and heart rate 88 bpm. The PMI is difficult to palpate secondary to her body size. Heart sounds are distant, but a low-pitched diastolic murmur is heard at the apex. Echocardiography is technically difficult, but LV function appears normal. Left atrium is mildly enlarged. Transvalvular mean mitral gradient is 5 mm Hg. By pressure half-time, the mitral valve area is estimated at 1.6 cm^2. There is mild mitral regurgitation. RV systolic pressure is 45 mm Hg. The next most appropriate step is:
    A. TEE
    B. Percutaneous mitral balloon valvotomy
    C. Mitral valve replacement
    D. Exercise testing with hemodynamic measurements
    E. Right and left cardiac catheterization

95. A 40-year-old male presents to hospital with transient dysarthria. Symptom duration was 90 minutes. The symptoms developed acutely on the morning of presentation while he was getting ready for work. He has no significant past medical history. He smokes one pack of cigarettes per day. He exercises regularly, jogging 1–2 miles several times per week. He denies any cardiac symptoms such as chest pain, dyspnea on exertion, or palpitations. Examination shows a BP of 132/80 mm Hg, and pulse is 70 bpm and regular. S_1 is accentuated, and an opening snap is heard approximately 0.10 seconds after A_2. A low-pitched diastolic murmur is also noted. A TEE is requested by the neurology service to exclude a cardiac source of emboli. This demonstrates normal LV and RV chamber sizes with normal systolic function. There is moderate biatrial enlargement. The interatrial septum is intact by color flow imaging and saline contrast study. There is doming of the anterior leaflet of the mitral valve in diastole. Mild commissural fusion is noted with just a few scattered areas of brightness at the leaflet margins consistent with calcification. Mitral valve area by planimetry is 1.4 cm². There is mild mitral regurgitation and mild tricuspid regurgitation. RV systolic pressure is estimated to be 40 mm Hg, and 48-hour Holter monitoring does not reveal any arrhythmias. For further treatment in this patient, you recommend:
    A. Aspirin 325 mg/day
    B. Aspirin 81 mg/day
    C. Clopidogrel 75 mg/day
    D. Aspirin/dipyridamole, one capsule b.i.d.
    E. Warfarin, with a goal INR of 2–3

96. A 55-year-old male is referred for evaluation of a heart murmur. He states that his family physician noted he had a murmur when he was in high school. It hadn't been mentioned again until he presented to his internist for a routine physical. He has a history of hypertension and paroxysmal atrial fibrillation, with two documented episodes in the past 3 years. The last episode lasted 12 hours, and he spontaneously converted. His medications include extended-release metoprolol 50 mg/day, hydrochlorothiazide 25 mg/day, and aspirin 81 mg/day. He is asymptomatic and exercises several times per week. Examination reveals a BP of 126/72 mm Hg and a pulse of 55 bpm. He has a systolic click and a grade III/VI holosystolic murmur at his apex. Echocardiography confirms your diagnosis of mitral valve prolapse with moderate mitral regurgitation. At this time, the next most appropriate recommendation is:
    A. No change in therapy; return for follow-up in 3 years
    B. No change in therapy; return for follow-up in 1 year
    C. Initiation of chronic anticoagulation
    D. Increase aspirin to 325 mg/day

97. Which of the following conditions is associated with bidirectional VT?
    A. Magnesium deficiency
    B. Hyperkalemia
    C. Metabolic acidosis
    D. Digoxin toxicity
    E. Lidocaine overdose

98. A 76-year-old female is hospitalized after an episode of syncope. She has a history of hypertension, hypothyroidism, hyperlipidemia, and osteoporosis. Her ECG shows sinus bradycardia at a rate of 44 bpm. Her QTc is 440 msec, and BP is 156/76 mm Hg. She is alert and oriented and denies any symptoms. Ten minutes after you examine her, the nurse calls and reports that the patient had an episode of transient loss of consciousness of <30 seconds in duration. On review of the telemetry, you note approximately 20 seconds of torsades de pointes that correlates with her symptoms. Currently, she is again bradycardic at a rate of 38 bpm. Your next action is to:
    A. Administer I.V. magnesium sulfate
    B. Administer I.V. amiodarone bolus and begin an infusion
    C. Administer I.V. procainamide
    D. Place transvenous pacemaker and administer I.V. beta-blocker
    E. Administer I.V. calcium gluconate

99. All of the following are considered major risk factors for sudden cardiac death in HCM EXCEPT:
    A. Nonsustained spontaneous VT
    B. Unexplained syncope
    C. High-risk mutation
    D. LV thickness ≥ 30 mm

100. A 74-year-old female is transferred from an outlying small town to your facility for further management. She has a history of hypothyroidism, breast cancer, and chronic kidney disease. She presented to the outlying facility complaining of dyspnea on minimal exertion. She also admits to orthopnea and nocturnal coughing over the past 3 days. On examination, she is alert, oriented, and answers questions appropriately. Her BP is 116/68 mm Hg, pulse 138 bpm and irregular, and respiratory rate 20. Her oxygen saturation is 86% on room air and 94% on 4 L of oxygen. Her jugular venous pulsation is elevated to the angle of her jaw. She has a grade II/VI systolic ejection murmur. Crackles are heard in the lower one third of her lung fields bilaterally. An ECG shows atrial fibrillation with rapid ventricular response and minor ST-segment and T-wave changes. The emergency department physician in the rural hospital has administered a 10 mg diltiazem bolus without a drip, 40 mg of I.V. furosemide, and 2 baby aspirin. After your examination, you elect to:

A. Administer an esmolol bolus and begin a drip
B. Sedate the patient and perform a direct current cardioversion
C. Administer an I.V. bolus of heparin, sedate the patient, and then perform a cardioversion
D. Administer an amiodarone bolus slowly and then begin an amiodarone drip
E. Administer another 10 mg bolus of diltiazem and then begin a continuous infusion. Add digoxin if her heart rate is not under control in 2 hours.

BOARD REVIEW ANSWERS

1. **C.** Patients with a bicuspid aortic valve have defects in the media, contributing to a higher prevalence of concomitant ascending aortic aneurysms. In addition, these patients' aneurysms expand at a faster rate compared to those in patients without a bicuspid aortic valve. Therefore, it is recommended that once the ascending aorta reaches 4 cm, the patient undergo annual imaging. Echocardiography is noninvasive and is the least expensive of the imaging modalities, but if the ascending aorta is not well visualized on echocardiography, CT or MRI should be performed.
(See Tadros TM, et al: Ascending aortic dilatation associated with bicuspid aortic valve: pathophysiology, molecular biology, and clinical implications, *Circulation* 119(6):880–890, 2009; and Hiratzka LF, et al: 2010 ACCF/AHA/AATS/ACR/ASA/SCA/SCAI/SIR/STS/SVM guidelines for the diagnosis and management of patients with thoracic aortic disease, *J Am Coll Cardiol* 55:1509–1544, 2010.)

2. **D.** A patient with a bicuspid aortic valve and an ascending aortic aneurysm should undergo elective repair when the aneurysm measures >4.5 cm if any of the following is also present: aortic coarctation whether or not it has been corrected, expansion rate of >0.5 cm/year (in an adult), first-degree relative with ascending aortic dissection or rupture, long smoking history with COPD. In addition, repair of the aorta is recommended when the aortic diameter is >4.5 cm if the adult patient is small and meets one of the following parameters: ratio of aortic area to body height > 10 cm^2/m or ratio of aortic diameter to BSA > 4.25 cm/m^2. (These are proposed guidelines suggested for use until validated in future research or studies.) Otherwise, elective repair is recommended when the aorta measures >5 cm in diameter or is >4 cm in diameter and the patient is undergoing aortic valve replacement.
(See Tadros TM, et al: Ascending aortic dilatation associated with bicuspid aortic valve: pathophysiology, molecular biology, and clinical implications, *Circulation* 119(6):880–890, 2009; and Hiratzka LF, et al: 2010 ACCF/AHA/AATS/ACR/ASA/SCA/SCAI/SIR/STS/SVM guidelines for the diagnosis and management of patients with thoracic aortic disease, *J Am Coll Cardiol* 55:1509–1544, 2010.)

3. **C.** The risk of aortic rupture, dissection, or aorta-related death markedly increases when the aortic aneurysm measures >6 cm in diameter. However, in patients with a bicuspid aortic valve, the aorta often dilates at a younger age and at a faster rate than in patients with normal aortic valve structure. Bicuspid aortic valve disease is associated with a ninefold higher lifetime risk of aortic dissection than in the general population. For idiopathic ascending aortic aneurysms, repair is recommended when the diameter reaches >5.5 cm. In patients with bicuspid aortic valve disease, repair is recommended when the aortic diameter is >5 cm because of the faster growth rate; the aneurysms may rupture at a younger patient age.
(See Tadros TM, et al: Ascending aortic dilatation associated with bicuspid aortic valve: pathophysiology, molecular biology, and clinical implications, *Circulation* 119(6):880–890, 2009; and Hiratzka LF, et al: 2010 ACCF/AHA/AATS/ACR/ASA/SCA/SCAI/SIR/STS/SVM guidelines for the diagnosis and management of patients with thoracic aortic disease, *J Am Coll Cardiol* 55:1509–1544, 2010.)

4. **C.** Surgical repair is recommended at an aortic diameter of 5.5 cm in patients with idiopathic ascending aortic aneurysms. This stems from the finding that aneurysms > 6 cm in diameter have a markedly increased risk of dissection or rupture.
(See Tadros TM, et al: Ascending aortic dilatation associated with bicuspid aortic valve: pathophysiology, molecular biology, and clinical implications, *Circulation* 119(6):880–890, 2009; and Hiratzka LF, et al: 2010 ACCF/AHA/AATS/ACR/ASA/SCA/SCAI/SIR/STS/SVM guidelines for the diagnosis and management of patients with thoracic aortic disease, *J Am Coll Cardiol* 55:1509–1544, 2010.)

5. **B.** In patients with congenital heart disease, atrial tachycardia is the most common arrhythmia. The mechanism most often involves a macroreentrant circuit within abnormal atrial tissue or muscle. This arrhythmia is termed IART. The reentrant rhythm may arise around incisions, scars, patches or other abnormal tissue. The rate is usually slower than in atrial flutter, often 150–250/min. Even though the arrhythmia may develop because of the congenital defect itself, more commonly the arrhythmia occurs secondary to prior surgeries intended to correct or palliate the congenital defect.
(See Walsh EP: Interventional electrophysiology in patients with congenital heart disease, *Circulation* 115:3224–3234, 2007.)

6. **D.** VT is a common arrhythmia in patients with tetralogy of Fallot. The prevalence has been estimated as being between 3% and 14%. The risk of sudden death has been estimated at approximately 2% per 10 years of follow-up. Some clinical factors that may indicate increased risk include older age at corrective surgery and at follow-up, history of prior shunt procedures, high-grade ventricular ectopy on Holter monitoring, inducible VT during EP study, prolonged duration of the QRS on ECG, and abnormal right heart size or function. When patients with tetralogy of Fallot develop significant arrhythmias, care should be taken to re-evaluate cardiac structures and function, including the pulmonic valve. The pulmonic valve may need repair or replacement if significant stenosis or regurgitation is found. However, this does not obviate the need for ICD placement in these patients because the incidence of VT or death has not been shown to decrease after valve surgery.
(See Walsh EP: Interventional electrophysiology in patients with congenital heart disease, *Circulation* 115:3224–3234, 2007; and Harrild DM, et al: Pulmonary valve replacement in tetralogy of Fallot: impact on survival and ventricular tachycardia, *Circulation* 119:445–451, 2009.)

7. **B.** An ASD is the most common concomitant structural cardiac abnormality in patients with Ebstein anomaly. All the other anomalies listed have been associated with Ebstein anomaly, but 80% to 94% of patients with Ebstein anomaly also have an ASD.
(See Attenhofer Jost CH, et al: Ebstein's anomaly, *Circulation* 115:277–285, 2007.)

8. **A.** First-degree AV block occurs in approximately 42% of patients with Ebstein anomaly. This may be because of RAE and abnormalities of the AV node. Complete heart block is uncommon in these patients. It has been estimated that 6% to 36% of Ebstein patients have one or more accessory pathways; as many as 20% may have WPW syndrome. The majority of the accessory pathways occur around the abnormal tricuspid valve. Atrial fibrillation and atrial flutter may also occur secondary to changes in the atrial myocardium, often secondary to previous surgery or atrial enlargement.
(See Attenhofer Jost CH, et al: Ebstein's anomaly, *Circulation* 115:277–285, 2007; and Walsh EP: Interventional electrophysiology in patients with congenital heart disease, *Circulation* 115:3224–3234, 2007.)

9. **C.** Rubella infection during the first trimester of pregnancy is associated with a high incidence of PDA. The incidence of PDA in children born at term is estimated at 1 in 2000 births, accounting for 5% to 10% of all congenital heart disease. The male to female ratio is estimated at 1:2. PDA occurs with increased frequency in many genetic syndromes, such as Down syndrome, Carpenter syndrome, and Holt-Oram syndrome, as well as several others.
(See Schneider DJ, Moore JW: Patent ductus arteriosus, *Circulation* 114:1873–1882, 2006.)

10. **C.** This patient has infective endarteritis of a PDA with septic emboli to the lungs, resulting in hypoxia, cough, and diminished breath sounds. The incidence of infective endarteritis in patients with PDA has decreased significantly; this decrease is attributed to surgical closure of the defect and use of antibiotics. Before these measures were common, the incidence was estimated at 1%/year and remains high in areas of the world with limited health care. Vegetations usually develop on the PA side of the ductus, resulting in pulmonary emboli. In this patient, blood cultures should be obtained to try and isolate a pathogen. A TEE or TTE should be completed to evaluate for a PDA. A PDA may be difficult to identify on a TTE because of the patient's body habitus, anatomy, or because of imaging difficulties. If PDA is suspected and not seen on TTE, a TEE should be completed. A CT of the chest with contrast should be completed to evaluate for embolic phenomenon to the lungs.
(See Schneider DJ, Moore JW: Patent ductus arteriosus, *Circulation* 114:1873–1882, 2006.)

11. **C**
(See Sommer RJ, et al: Pathophysiology of congenital heart disease in the adult: part III: complex congenital heart disease, *Circulation* 117:1340–1350, 2008.)

12. **E**
(See Sommer RJ, et al: Pathophysiology of congenital heart disease in the adult: part III: complex congenital heart disease, *Circulation* 117:1340–1350, 2008.)

13. **A**
(See Sommer RJ, et al: Pathophysiology of congenital heart disease in the adult: part III: complex congenital heart disease, *Circulation* 117:1340–1350, 2008.)

14. **F**
(See Sommer RJ, et al: Pathophysiology of congenital heart disease in the adult: part III: complex congenital heart disease, *Circulation* 117:1340–1350, 2008.)

15. **D**
(See Sommer RJ, et al: Pathophysiology of congenital heart disease in the adult: part III: complex congenital heart disease, *Circulation* 117:1340–1350, 2008.)

16. **B**
(See Sommer RJ, et al: Pathophysiology of congenital heart disease in the adult: part III: complex congenital heart disease, *Circulation* 117:1340–1350, 2008.)

17. **B** and **C**
(See Sommer RJ, et al: Pathophysiology of congenital heart disease in the adult: part III: complex congenital heart disease, *Circulation* 117:1340–1350, 2008.)

18. **D**
(See Sommer RJ, et al: Pathophysiology of congenital heart disease in the adult: part III: complex congenital heart disease, *Circulation* 117:1340–1350, 2008.)

19. **A**
(See Sommer RJ, et al: Pathophysiology of congenital heart disease in the adult: part III: complex congenital heart disease, *Circulation* 117:1340–1350, 2008.)

20. **A**
(See Sommer RJ, et al: Pathophysiology of congenital heart disease in the adult: part III: complex congenital heart disease, *Circulation* 117:1340–1350, 2008.)

21. **C.** When a Fontan patient presents with significant symptoms of right heart failure or cyanosis, evaluation in the cardiac catheterization laboratory is commonly needed to identify the site of concern. Small pressure gradients across the constructed venous structures may indicate a significant resistance to flow and may not be readily apparent on noninvasive imaging. Obstruction may be found in the PA branches or at suture lines and can be dilated by balloon catheters if identified. Embolization of any collaterals that have formed between the aorta and PA can also be completed. Angiographic evaluation of the Fontan pathway is especially useful in patients with cyanosis. It may help identify intracardiac shunts or venous collaterals. After careful consideration, these may be closed or embolized, but at times symptoms may worsen because of the elimination of the right-to-left shunt. Care of these patients is often difficult and complex, and evaluation in the catheterization laboratory by experienced operators is extremely useful.
(See Sommer RJ, et al: Pathophysiology of congenital heart disease in the adult: part III: complex congenital heart disease, *Circulation* 117:1340–1350, 2008.)

22. **E.** The patient is a diabetic; therefore, his goal BP is <130/80 mm Hg. The most reasonable approach is to titrate his ramipril to the maximum dose before adding an additional medication or switching to another medication. An ARB or direct renin inhibitor is not more beneficial than an ACE inhibitor in diabetic patients. Adding hydrochlorothiazide in a combination pill would be reasonable once his current medication has been maximized. Adding a beta-blocker is a possibility but is not the best choice given his pulse is 65 bpm and this would be adding another pill.
(See Chobanian AV, et al: The seventh report of the Joint National Committee on Prevention, Detection, Evaluation, and Treatment of High Blood Pressure: the JNC 7 report, *JAMA* 289:2560–2571, 2003.)

23. **C.** In patients with high triglyceride levels (200–499 mg/dL), it is recommended that a patient's non-HDL cholesterol be <130 mg/dL; further reduction to <100 mg/dL is reasonable. LDL-lowering therapy should be used first before prescribing additional agents such as niacin or fibrates. Non-HDL cholesterol is calculated as

$$TC - HDL = \text{non-HDL cholesterol}$$

LDL is calculated by the formula:

$$LDL = TC - (\text{triglycerides} / 5 - HDL)$$

However, this calculation is inaccurate when the triglycerides are elevated.
(See Fraker TD Jr, Fihn SD: 2007 chronic angina focused update of the ACC/AHA 2002 guidelines for the management of patients with chronic stable angina, *J Am Coll Cardiol* 50(23):2264–2274, 2007.)

24. **D.** Nicotinic acid inhibits mobilization of free fatty acids from peripheral tissues, thereby reducing hepatic synthesis of triglycerides and VLDL secretion. Niacin may increase HDL by as much as 30% and is currently the most effective medication available to increase HDL levels. The main adverse effect of niacin is flushing, which is prostaglandin mediated and may be reduced by taking aspirin approximately 30 minutes before the niacin dose. In addition, niacin may raise blood glucose levels; therefore, cautious use and close follow-up is recommended in diabetic patients. Uric acid levels may also increase; therefore, it is not recommended in patients with gout.
(See Lenfant C, et al: Seventh report of the Joint National Committee on the Prevention, Detection, Evaluation, and Treatment of High Blood Pressure (JNC 7): resetting the hypertension sails, *Hypertension* 41:1178–1179, 2003.)
(See Rader DJ: Effects of nonstatin lipid drug therapy on high-density lipoprotein metabolism, *Am J Cardiol* 91:e18–e23, 2003.)

25. **B.** It is thought that hypothyroidism may lead to increased LDL levels because of down-regulation of the LDL receptor and an increased half-life of LDL cholesterol because of decreased metabolism. In a previously controlled patient, one should suspect hypothyroidism as an etiology of markedly increased lipid levels. This patient has gained weight, is bradycardic, and complains of increased fatigue, which all may be secondary to hypothyroidism.
(See Cappola AR, Ladenson PW: Hypothyroidism and atherosclerosis, *J Clin Endocrinol Metab* 88:2438–2444, 2003.)

26. **A.** The ACC/AHA give a class I recommendation to tricuspid valve repair at the time of mitral valve surgery in a patient with severe tricuspid regurgitation. It is less clear how to proceed in patients with less than severe tricuspid regurgitation. It is a class IIb recommendation for repair in less than severe tricuspid regurgitation. However, it has been suggested that patients with moderate tricuspid regurgitation or tricuspid annular dilatation > 40 mm undergo repair of the tricuspid valve at the time of mitral valve surgery. It is known that patient outcome is poor for patients requiring tricuspid valve surgery after having undergone mitral valve surgery in the past. This patient had tricuspid valve annular dilatation (malcoaptation of the tricuspid leaflets, which appeared normal) with severe tricuspid regurgitation; therefore, the patient should undergo repair of the tricuspid valve at the time of her mitral valve replacement. This patient has severe mitral stenosis, signified by the gradient of 12 mm Hg, and at least moderate mitral regurgitation and therefore is not a candidate for mitral valve balloon valvotomy.
(See Shiran A, Sagie A: Tricuspid regurgitation in mitral valve disease incidence, prognostic implications, mechanism, and management, *J Am Coll Cardiol* 53:401–408, 2009.)

27. **C.** The DAVID trial demonstrated that patients who had their dual-chamber ICD programmed to a dual-chamber rate-adaptive mode at 70 bpm had increased risk of the primary endpoint, heart failure hospitalization, and mortality compared to patients with their device programmed to single-chamber pacing at 40 bpm. The negative effects of DDDR pacing was thought to be secondary to RV pacing; therefore, many now try to minimize RV pacing.
(See Wilkoff BL, et al: Dual-chamber pacing or ventricular backup pacing in patients with an implantable defibrillator: the Dual Chamber and VVI Implantable Defibrillator (DAVID) Trial, *JAMA* 288:3115–3123, 2002.)

28. **B.** In moyamoya patients, stenosis and narrowing occurs in the distal ICA and may also involve the proximal anterior and middle cerebral arteries. The narrowing is not due to an atherosclerotic process, but rather is secondary to smooth muscle cell hyperplasia and thrombosis of the lumens of the arteries. Collaterals develop that are fragile and prone to hemorrhage. Dilated collaterals are also thought to be responsible for the headaches the patients often experience. Ischemic symptoms or stroke occurs in the regions of decreased blood flow. Radiation to the head and neck is a risk factor for the development of moyamoya disease. Angiography provides a definitive diagnosis with a characteristic appearance of the distal ICA and the proximal anterior and middle cerebral arteries. An extensive collateral network and "puff of smoke" appearance of collaterals may also be seen. Treatment most often consists of surgery using the spared ECA to directly or indirectly supply blood to the ischemic regions of the brain. WAGR syndrome is hypertension associated with Wilms' tumor.
(See Scott RM, Smith ER: Moyamoya disease and moyamoya syndrome, *N Engl J Med* 360:1226–1237, 2009.)

29. **D.** The OPTIC trial was a secondary prevention trial in patients with spontaneous or inducible VT; 38.5% of patients on beta-blockers experienced a defibrillator shock, 24.3% of patients on sotalol experienced a shock, and 10.3% of patients on a combination of amiodarone and a beta-blocker experienced a defibrillator shock.
(See Connolly SJ, et al: Comparison of beta-blockers, amiodarone plus beta-blockers, or sotalol for prevention of shocks from implantable cardioverter defibrillators: the OPTIC Study: a randomized trial, *JAMA* 295:165–167, 2006.)

30. **E.** In asymptomatic athletes, the AHA recommends preparticipation history and physical examination. Routine ECG screening in athletes has been in place in Italy for many years and has recently been advocated by the European Society of Cardiology.
(See Maron BJ, et al: Recommendations and considerations related to preparticipation screening for cardiovascular abnormalities in competitive athletes: 2007 update, *Circulation* 115:1643–1655, 2007; and Corrado D, et al: Pre-participation screening of young competitive athletes for prevention of sudden cardiac death, *J Am Coll Cardiol* 52:1981–1989, 2008.)

31. **C.** The patient has no evidence of residual heart disease by clinical examination or echocardiogram. She should receive prophylaxis for 10 years or until age 21, whichever is longer. The agent recommended in most instances is I.M. benzathine penicillin every 4 weeks. The alternative is oral penicillin V 250 mg b.i.d. If this patient did have clinical or echocardiographic evidence of rheumatic heart disease (persistent valvular disease), prophylaxis is then recommended until age 40 or for 10 years, whichever is longer. If a patient has rheumatic fever without carditis, prophylaxis is recommended for 5 years or until age 21, whichever is longer.
(See Gerber MA, et al: Prevention of rheumatic fever and diagnosis and treatment of acute streptococcal pharyngitis, *Circulation* 119:1541–1551, 2009.)

32. **B.** Candesartan was studied in the Candesartan in Heart Failure: Assessment of Reduction in Mortality and Morbidity (CHARM) series of research studies. It was shown that candesartan reduces cardiovascular death and hospitalizations from heart failure (NYHA class II–IV, ejection fraction $\leq$ 40%). In addition it may have added benefit when used with an ACE inhibitor in heart failure treatment regimens (CHARM-Added trial).
(See Granger CB, et al: Effects of candesartan in patients with chronic heart failure and reduced left-ventricular systolic function intolerant to angiotensin-converting-enzyme inhibitors: the CHARM-Alternative trial, *Lancet* 362(9386):772–776, 2003.)

33. **D.** It is recommended that patients diagnosed with idiopathic venous thromboembolism undergo a complete history and physical examination. In addition routine laboratory tests, chest x-ray, and age- and sex-specific cancer screening is reasonable. Additional screening can be completed based on the patient's risk factors and clinical findings. To date, there is no firm evidence to support an extensive work-up or screening regimen to detect occult malignancy in patients with idiopathic venous thromboembolism.
(See Mickelson D, et al: A 43-year-old woman with chest pressure, *Cleve Clin J Med* 76:191–198, 2009.)

34. **E.** In the past, colchicine was recommended as treatment for recurrent episodes of pericarditis. However, in the Colchicine for Acute Pericarditis (COPE) trial, colchicine was also found to be beneficial for first episodes of acute pericarditis. In this trial, patients treated with aspirin and colchicine had reduced rates of recurrent episodes of pericarditis. Aspirin, indomethacin, or ibuprofen are the medications most often prescribed with colchicine. 0.5–1 mg of colchicine is recommended daily. The European Society of Cardiology guidelines on the Diagnosis and Management of Pericardial Diseases recommend colchicine 0.5 mg b.i.d. for the initial treatment of acute pericarditis (class IIa, level of evidence: B).
(See Imazio M, et al: Colchicine in addition to conventional therapy for acute pericarditis: results of the COlchicine for acute PEricarditis (COPE) trial, *Circulation* 112:2012–2016, 2005; and Maisch B, et al: Guidelines on the diagnosis and management of pericardial diseases, *Eur Heart J* 25:587–610, 2004.)

35. **D.** Myxomas are the most common primary cardiac tumors. They are benign and most often arise in the left atrium. The mean age at presentation is 50 years; two thirds of patients are female. Papillary fibroelastomas are the most common tumors of the cardiac valves and are most often found on the aortic and mitral valves. Fibroelastomas most often occur singly. Sarcomas are the most common malignant neoplasms of the heart. Lipomas are rare.
(See Sabatine MS, et al: Primary tumors of the heart. In Zipes DP, et al, editors: *Braunwald's Heart Disease: A Textbook of Cardiovascular Medicine*, ed 7, Philadelphia, 2005, Elsevier, pp 1741–1757.)

36. **A.** Approximately 25% of all cardiac tumors are malignant; it is estimated that 95% of these are sarcomas. Angiosarcoma is the most common type of sarcoma arising in the heart, often arising in the right atrium. Patients often present late, after the tumor has metastasized. In addition, patients often present with right-sided heart failure. If the tumor is infiltrative, it may extend into the pericardium, causing a pericardial effusion. Surgical resection is the preferred treatment but may be difficult if the tumor is infiltrative. Chemotherapy or radiotherapy is used for metastases but is usually not curative. Median survival in these patients is 6–12 months, with increased median survival in those able to undergo complete excision.
(See Sabatine MS, et al: Primary tumors of the heart. In Zipes DP, et al, editors: *Braunwald's Heart Disease: A Textbook of Cardiovascular Medicine*, ed 7, Philadelphia, 2005, Elsevier, pp 1741–1757.)

37. **D.** The AHA recommends that people consume fatty fish two times per week. Patients with CAD should consume 1 gram of EPA and DHA per day. In patients with hypertriglyceridemia, fish oil supplements can be used to help lower triglyceride levels. HDL levels may also increase. LDL levels have been shown to increase slightly, averaging 10 mg/dL in one review. There is some data to support the contention that the combination of a statin and fish oil supplements may reduce the risk of coronary events. Lovaza, a combination of EPA and DHA, is approved by the FDA for the treatment of hypertriglyceridemia, levels > 500 mg/dL. The recommended dose is 2–4 g/day.
(See Chan EJ, Cho L: What can we expect from omega-3 fatty acids, *Cleve Clin J Med* 76:245–251, 2009.)

38. **B.** In the ACUITY trial, there were three arms: bivalirudin alone, UFH/enoxaparin + glycoprotein IIb/IIIa inhibitor, or bivalirudin + glycoprotein IIb/IIIa inhibitor. There was no difference in ischemic endpoints between the three arms. However, there was a statistically significant lower rate of major bleeding in the bivalirudin alone (4%) arm versus the UFH/enoxaparin + glycoprotein IIb/IIIa inhibitor (7%) and bivalirudin + glycoprotein IIb/IIIa inhibitor (8%) arms.
(See Dixon SR, et al: The year in interventional cardiology, *J Am Coll Cardiol* 51:2355–2369, 2008; and Stone GW, et al: Bivalirudin for patients with acute coronary syndromes, *N Engl J Med* 355:2203–2216, 2006.)

39. **C.** The 10-year results of the BARI trial showed no difference in mortality between PCI and CABG patients. However, in the subgroup of diabetic patients, there was lower mortality in those undergoing CABG compared to PCI. The BARI trial did not compare medical therapy to PCI or CABG.
(See Dixon SR, et al: The year in interventional cardiology, *J Am Coll Cardiol* 51:2355–2369, 2008; and BARI Investigators: The final 10-year follow-up results from the BARI randomized trial, *J Am Coll Cardiol* 49:1600–1606, 2007.)

40. **C.** This patient has class IV CHF with multiple admissions in the past 6 months. She has signs and symptoms of congestion but not of organ hypoperfusion. Therefore, continuous I.V. inotrope is not indicated; intermittent infusion of inotropes is a class III recommendation. Use of Swan-Ganz catheters in the management of heart failure is limited. It may be indicated in the following situations: in a patient thought to have cardiogenic shock, in a patient with signs of hypoperfusion and whose filling pressures are difficult to determine clinically, in a patient dependent on inotrope therapy despite clinical improvement, and in a patient with continued severe symptoms despite adjustments in therapy. Spironolactone should not be added to her regimen because of her renal dysfunction (elevated serum Cr). The patient should not be placed in a long-term care facility without first openly discussing this option with her and her family. The patient's prognosis is poor and end-of-life options, including turning off her defibrillator, should be openly discussed with her and her family. In patients with end-stage, refractory heart failure, discussing end-of-life plans and the option of turning off the defibrillator is a class I recommendation.
(See Jessup M, et al: 2009 focused update: ACCF/AHA Guidelines for the Diagnosis and Management of Heart Failure in Adults, *Circulation* 119:1977–2016, 2009.)

41. **C.** Adding a fixed-dose combination of isosorbide mononitrate and hydralazine to standard heart failure therapy is a class I recommendation for African American patients. Bisoprolol, long-acting metoprolol, or carvedilol are all reasonable beta-blockers to use in patients with heart failure. There is no solid data to support using an ARB over an ACE inhibitor in heart failure, although an ARB can be added to an ACE inhibitor in patients with heart failure and may be of some benefit (class IIb recommendation). Placing a Holter monitor to detect arrhythmia is low yield in this patient. However, prophylactic ICD placement for primary prevention would be indicated. Isolated mitral valve repair in ischemic cardiomyopathy is not recommended. However, it is reasonable to perform mitral valve annuloplasty in patients with significant mitral regurgitation at the time of CABG.
(See Jessup M, et al: 2009 focused update: ACCF/AHA Guidelines for the Diagnosis and Management of Heart Failure in Adults, *Circulation* 119:1977–2016, 2009.)

42. **D.** Spironolactone should not be added to the medication regimen of a patient on an ACE inhibitor and an ARB (class III recommendation). It would be beneficial to add spironolactone if the patient were taking either an ACE inhibitor or ARB, but not both. This patient is a candidate for ICD placement but not biventricular pacing, which requires a QRS duration of >120 msec. His is 118 msec. Currently, this is the only method used in the guidelines to measure dyssynchrony. Imaging parameters are still being investigated but are not currently approved to define dyssynchrony. This patient has not been hospitalized for >1 year; therefore, digoxin is not the best choice in this scenario. Digoxin has been shown to decrease heart failure admissions but not mortality. Increasing the patient's furosemide dose is also not the best choice; he does not have signs or symptoms of significant congestion. The best answer is to titrate up his carvedilol. In clinical trials, carvedilol has been shown to decrease mortality in the heart failure population.
(See Jessup M, et al: 2009 focused update: ACCF/AHA Guidelines for the Diagnosis and Management of Heart Failure in Adults, *Circulation* 119:1977–2016, 2009.)

43. **B.** Absolute indications for cardiac transplant in appropriate patients include those with refractory cardiogenic shock, dependence on I.V. inotrope therapy to maintain adequate organ perfusion, peak VO_2 < 10 mL/kg/min with achievement of anaerobic metabolism, severe symptoms of ischemia that consistently limit daily activities in those whose anatomy is not amenable to intervention (CABG or PCI), and recurrent symptomatic ventricular arrhythmias refractory to all therapeutic modalities. Relative indications include peak VO_2 11–14 mL/kg/min with significant limitation in patient's daily activity, recurrent unstable ischemia not amenable to other intervention, and recurrent instability of fluid balance/kidney function in a patient compliant with the medical regimen. Insufficient indications include severely depressed LV ejection fraction, functional class III–IV CHF, and peak VO_2 >15 mL/kg/min without other indications.
(See Hunt SA, et al: 2009 focused update incorporated into the ACC/AHA 2005 guidelines for the diagnosis and management of heart failure in adults, *Circulation* 119:e391–e479, 2009.)

44. **D.** Early afterdepolarizations can occur when there is net positivity intracellularly. Early afterdepolarizations may prolong the action potential, resulting in ventricular arrhythmias and torsades de pointes. Hypokalemia, hypomagnesemia, and increased catecholamines may contribute to early afterdepolarizations. Drugs such as sotalol, N-acetylprocainamide, and quinidine may contribute to early afterdepolarizations. Delayed afterdepolarizations may be related to the accumulation of intracellular calcium. Some of the arrhythmias precipitated by digoxin may be due to delayed afterdepolarizations.
(See Rubart M, Zipes DP: Genesis of cardiac arrhythmias: electrophysiological considerations. In Zipes DP, et al, editors: *Braunwald's Heart Disease: A Textbook of Cardiovascular Medicine*, ed 7, Philadelphia, 2005, Elsevier, pp 653–687.)

45. **D.** Ibutilide is a class III antiarrhythmic medication used intravenously to convert atrial fibrillation or flutter to sinus rhythm. It is given as a rapid infusion of 1 mg over 10 minutes. It should not be used if the QTc is >440 msec or if hypokalemia or bradycardia is present. Torsades de pointes occurs in 2% of patients who receive the drug. Patients should be monitored for at least 6 hours after its administration. None of the other listed medicines are approved for I.V. use to acutely convert atrial fibrillation or flutter.
(See Miller JM, Zipes DP: Therapy for cardiac arrhythmias. In Zipes DP, et al, editors: *Braunwald's Heart Disease: A Textbook of Cardiovascular Medicine*, ed 7, Philadelphia, 2005, Elsevier, pp 713–766.)

46. **A.** The defibrillation threshold is increased by most antiarrhythmic medications, particularly those that alter sodium channel conductance, such as class I drugs and amiodarone. On the other hand, sotalol may decrease the frequency of ICD shocks and decrease the defibrillation threshold.
(See Miller JM, Zipes DP: Therapy for cardiac arrhythmias. In Zipes DP, et al, editors: *Braunwald's Heart Disease: A Textbook of Cardiovascular Medicine*, ed 7, Philadelphia, 2005, Elsevier, pp 713–766.)

47. **B.** Performing exercise ECG can help risk-stratify this patient. If the patient's ECG normalizes during exercise, this indicates that the accessory pathway has a longer antegrade effective refractory period and the risk of sudden death is low compared to a patient with an accessory pathway with a shorter refractory period.
(See Olgin JE, Zipes DP: Specific arrhythmias: diagnosis and treatment. In Zipes DP, et al, editors: *Braunwald's Heart Disease: A Textbook of Cardiovascular Medicine*, ed 7, Philadelphia, 2005, Elsevier, pp 803–863.)

48. **D.** Brugada syndrome is caused by mutation of the cardiac sodium channel gene (*SCN5A*). The mutations identified cause a reduction in the sodium current. Long QT syndrome 3 is characterized by gain-of-function mutations of the cardiac sodium channel. The Na⁺ inward current increases, and the action potential is prolonged. Long QT syndrome 3 and long QT syndrome 2 are characterized by mutations that affect K⁺ channels.
(See Olgin JE, Zipes DP: Specific arrhythmias: diagnosis and treatment. In Zipes DP, et al, editor: *Braunwald's Heart Disease: A Textbook of Cardiovascular Medicine*, ed 7, Philadelphia, 2005, Elsevier, pp 803–863.)

49. **1, B. 2, A. 3, C. 4, C.** Long QT syndrome 1 is associated with sudden death during exercise, especially swimming. Long QT syndrome 2 is associated with sudden death after significant auditory stimuli, such as a loud alarm clock, or with emotional situations. Long QT syndrome 3 and Brugada syndrome are associated with sudden death occurring during rest or sleep.
(See Olgin JE, Zipes DP: Specific arrhythmias: diagnosis and treatment. In Zipes DP, et al, editor: *Braunwald's Heart Disease: A Textbook of Cardiovascular Medicine*, ed 7, Philadelphia, 2005, Elsevier, pp 803–863.)

50. **C.** In the STICH trial, CABG alone was compared to CABG plus SVR using various surgical techniques. After a follow-up of a median of 4 years, there was no statistically significant difference between the two arms in regard to the primary endpoint of all-cause mortality or cardiac rehospitalization. In addition there was no difference in symptoms or exercise tolerance between the groups.
(See Jones RH, et al: Coronary bypass surgery with or without surgical ventricular reconstruction, *N Engl J Med* 360:1705–1717, 2009.)

51. **C.** Neurocardiogenic syncope is the most common cause of syncope in young patients as well as middle-aged patients. Cough-, micturition-, deglutination-, and defecation-induced syncope, all forms of neurocardiogenic syncope, are more common in middle-aged or elderly patients. Elderly patients are also more likely to experience syncope from such things as aortic stenosis, pulmonary embolus, or arrhythmias secondary to co-existing heart disease.
(See Strickberger SA, et al: AHA/ACCF scientific statement on the evaluation of syncope, *Circulation* 113:316–327, 2006.)

52. **A.** The history is the most important step in the evaluation of syncope. History, not only from the patient, but also from any onlookers, is extremely important. The physical examination should focus on identifying the presence of structural heart disease. The cause of syncope remains elusive in approximately 40% of cases.
(See Strickberger SA, et al: AHA/ACCF scientific statement on the evaluation of syncope, *Circulation* 113:316–327, 2006: and Benditt DG, Nguyen JT: Syncope: therapeutic approaches, *J Am Coll Cardiol* 53:1741–1751, 2009.)

53. **D.** According to the AHA/ACCF Scientific Statement on the Evaluation of Syncope, published in 2006, exercise ECG should be completed in a patient with unexplained syncope and risk factors for CAD. In this case, if the stress test was normal, the evaluation would then be complete. If the patient has recurrent episodes, then a Holter monitor, event monitor, or implantable loop recorder could be considered. TIAs rarely result in syncope. However, patients with severe bilateral carotid disease may experience syncope. Tonic-clonic, seizure-like activity is seen in both cardiac and neurologic causes of syncope.
(See Strickberger SA, et al: AHA/ACCF scientific statement on the evaluation of syncope, *Circulation* 113:316–327, 2006.)

54. **A.** Adult and pediatric patients with severe LV failure within 2 weeks of a viral illness and lymphocytic myocarditis on EMB have an excellent prognosis. It is a class I indication to perform an EMB in patients with the above presentation. All of the other answers are true.
(See Cooper LT, et al: The role of endomyocardial biopsy in the management of cardiovascular disease, *Circulation* 116:2216–2233, 2007.)

55. **C.** GCM should be differentiated from cardiac sarcoidosis. Patients with GCM are usually white, whereas those with sarcoidosis are most often black. Patients with GCM have more rapid progression of their symptoms. Patients with sarcoidosis more often present with syncope and less severe CHF. Sarcoidosis patients have a better prognosis than those with GCM. Histologically both have giant cells, but only sarcoidosis has noncaseating granulomas present. In GCM, myocyte necrosis is usually present, but it is usually absent in sarcoidosis. Performing an EMB in a patient with new-onset heart failure of 2 weeks' to 3 months' duration associated with a dilated ventricle and new ventricular arrhythmias, second- or third-degree heart block, or failure to respond to usual care within 1–2 weeks is a class I indication. A predominantly lymphocytic infiltrate is seen in myocarditis occurring after a recent viral infection. A predominance of eosinophils with significant myocyte necrosis is typical of necrotizing eosinophilic myocarditis, a rare condition that is usually rapidly progressive and often fatal.
(See Cooper LT, et al: The role of endomyocardial biopsy in the management of cardiovascular disease, *Circulation* 116:2216–2233, 2007.)

56. **B.** GCM has a poor prognosis, with a mean transplantation-free survival of only 5.5 months. GCM is associated with thymoma and various autoimmune disorders. VT and heart block are commonly present in patients with GCM. Combination immunosuppressive therapy may increase transplantation-free survival. In one study, patients not receiving immunosuppressive therapy had a median survival of 3 months versus 12.3 months in those patients treated with combination immunosuppressive therapy. Heart transplantation is the mainstay of treatment for patients with GCM.
(See Cooper LT, et al: The role of endomyocardial biopsy in the management of cardiovascular disease, *Circulation* 116:2216–2233, 2007.)

57. **C.** The baroreceptor response is often decreased in elderly patients. In addition to the changes listed, the heart rate response to orthostatic stress is also often blunted in the elderly.
(See Strickberger SA, et al: AHA/ACCF scientific statement on the evaluation of syncope, *Circulation* 113:316–327, 2006.)

58. **C.** The patient should undergo an EP study because syncope occurring during exercise is suggestive of a primary arrhythmia or structural origin of syncope. This patient's echocardiogram and ischemia evaluation were normal. Therefore, a primary arrhythmia may be the reason for her syncope; an EP study may help determine this. Other clinical findings suggesting a cardiac cause of syncope include physical examination or echocardiographic evidence of severe structural heart disease, syncope while supine, palpitations at the time of syncope, history of heart failure, acute or prior MI, evidence of LV dysfunction, and certain abnormalities on the ECG. Some indications for an EP study to evaluate the cause of syncope include an abnormal ECG, suggesting conduction system disease, syncope during exercise or supine, syncope in patients with significant structural heart disease, syncope with palpitations or angina-like chest discomfort, and a family history of sudden death. The European Society of Cardiology published guidelines on the Evaluation and Treatment of Syncope in 2004. EP study is rated a class I indication for a patient experiencing syncope during exertion.
(See Benditt DG, Nguyen JT: Syncope: therapeutic approaches, *J Am Coll Cardiol* 53:1741–1751, 2009: and Brignole M, et al: Guidelines on management (diagnosis and treatment) of syncope—update 2004, *Eur Heart J* 25:2054–2072, 2004.)

59. **True.** According to the AHA/ACCF Scientific Statement on the Evaluation of Syncope, after an ischemic evaluation, patients with CAD and syncope should undergo an EP study. Regardless of the patient's LV function, patients with CAD, syncope, and inducible monomorphic VT during EP study should have a defibrillator placed.
(See Strickberger SA, et al: AHA/ACCF scientific statement on the evaluation of syncope, *Circulation* 113:316–327, 2006.)

60. **D.** AMI occurs at all stages of pregnancy. It is most common in patients over age 30 and in multigravid women. The anterior wall is the most common myocardial segment involved. In a review by Roth et al., coronary dissection accounted for the majority of cases of AMI in the peripartum period and was more common in the postpartum than in the antepartum period. Progesterone excess or eosinophilic inflammation is thought to possibly play a contributing role in spontaneous coronary artery dissections. Thrombolytic therapy is relatively contraindicated in pregnancy, but in this instance the patient is 6 weeks postpartum. Nonetheless, this patient has a high likelihood that spontaneous coronary artery dissection is the etiology of her AMI. Thrombolytic therapy may increase the risk of bleeding and propagation of the dissection. Coronary angiography is the best option in this patient's situation because of the high likelihood of coronary artery dissection. This patient should be started on heparin before transfer; it is thought that this may help maintain flow down the true arterial lumen. In addition, standard treatment for AMI, such as I.V. nitroglycerin and aspirin, is indicated. Even though spontaneous coronary artery dissection is most likely, there is still the possibility that her infarction is occurring from acute plaque rupture or thombotic occlusion of the coronary artery. At angiography, if flow in the dissected coronary artery is adequate to the distal vessel, it may be treated conservatively without stenting. Some reports indicate that if the dissection heals without intervention, the patient may have a more favorable outcome. However, if flow is compromised in the vessel, coronary intervention with stenting or, if necessary, CABG is undertaken. (See Roth A, Elkayam U: Acute myocardial infarction associated with pregnancy, *J Am Coll Cardiol* 52:171–180, 2008; and Almeda FQ, et al: Spontaneous coronary artery dissection, *Clin Cardiol* 27:377–380, 2004.)

61. **C.** This patient has developed a stress-related cardiomyopathy characterized by transient LV dysfunction. This is also known as *Takotsubo cardiomyopathy* or *apical ballooning syndrome*. Most often the apical (with or without midventricular) myocardial segments are significantly impaired. In addition, the basal segments may become hyperdynamic to compensate. This can lead to a dynamic outflow tract obstruction with or without SAM of the mitral valve. If SAM is present, significant mitral regurgitation may develop. These changes can contribute to the development of heart failure and malperfusion. (See Bybee KA, Prasad A: Stress-related cardiomyopathy syndromes, *Circulation* 118:397–409, 2008.)

62. **D.** This patient has begun to develop signs of hemodynamic compromise secondary to a dynamic outflow tract obstruction. Her BP is borderline low, and her heart rate is near the upper limits of normal. She has bilateral crackles secondary to pulmonary edema from heart failure. The mitral regurgitation is a result of SAM of the mitral valve. Treatment of this patient is similar to that of a patient with a similar clinical picture and HCM. If respiratory status allows, the patient should be given I.V. fluids. Intravenous beta-blockers should be administered to decrease the outflow tract obstruction by decreasing heart rate and contractility. Use of a pure alpha-blocker like phenylephrine may be tried if beta-blockers and fluids are not tolerated. It is also possible that patients with transient stress-induced myocardial dysfunction may have severely depressed LV function resulting in shock, requiring inotropic or IABP support. Eventually the patient will require furosemide therapy to treat the pulmonary edema, but currently she is oxygenating adequately; it is important to immediately try to decrease the outflow tract obstruction to prevent further hemodynamic compromise. Obtaining an echocardiogram is helpful to assess wall motion but should not be completed until the patient is stabilized. One may elect to perform a diagnostic cardiac catheterization in this patient, but again this should be performed after the patient is stabilized. (See Bybee KA, Prasad A: Stress-related cardiomyopathy syndromes, *Circulation* 118:397–409, 2008.)

63. **A.** In order of frequency, the most common ECG changes in patients with intracranial bleeding or ischemic stroke are QT-interval prolongation, ST-segment depression, and U waves. A prolonged QT interval is more often seen in patients with SAH than in patients with other intracranial pathology and may be the reason for increased risk of ventricular arrhythmias in these patients. If neurogenic stress cardiomyopathy occurs, transient ST-segment elevation may be noted. Often, if cardiomyopathy develops, deep symmetrical T-wave inversions develop. (See Bybee KA, Prasad A: Stress-related cardiomyopathy syndromes, *Circulation* 118:397–409, 2008.)

64. **D.** Postoperative atrial fibrillation is the most common complication encountered after cardiac surgery. The incidence of postoperative atrial fibrillation is 30% after CABG alone, 40% after valve surgery, and 50% after CABG and valve surgery combined. The peak incidence is on postoperative day 2. The most consistent predictor for the occurrence of postoperative atrial fibrillation is advanced age. The risk for perioperative stroke is three times higher for patients with postoperative atrial fibrillation. Beta-blockers should be administered to patients undergoing cardiac surgery to prevent postoperative atrial fibrillation unless contraindicated (class I, level of evidence: A). If beta-blockers cannot be given, amiodarone should be given preoperatively to patients at high risk of developing postoperative atrial fibrillation because it has been shown to reduce the incidence of atrial fibrillation in patients undergoing cardiac surgery (class IIa, level of evidence: B). Several trials have demonstrated the efficacy of amiodarone therapy, administered preoperatively as well as postoperatively, in preventing postoperative atrial fibrillation: Amiodarone Reduction in Coronary Heart (ARCH) trial and Prophylactic Oral Amiodarone for the Prevention of Arrhythmias that Begin Early After Revascularization, Valve Replacement, or Repair (PAPABEAR) trial. This patient is asthmatic and cannot be treated with a beta-blocker. His mitral regurgitation is not severe enough to require repair with an annuloplasty ring. He is at increased risk of postoperative atrial fibrillation. He has PACs on his ECG and moderate LAE. Amiodarone administered now and continued postoperatively would be appropriate to try and decrease his risk of developing atrial fibrillation. Adding a statin to the patient's regimen is important for him lifelong but isn't likely to provide as much immediate benefit as amiodarone therapy. A recent study—Atorvastatin for Reduction of Myocardial Dysrhythmia After Cardiac Surgery (ARMYDA-3)—showed that perioperative statin therapy reduces the incidence of postoperative atrial fibrillation. Tight blood glucose control is important in the postoperative period, but atrial fibrillation is the most common postoperative complication.
(See Echahidi N, et al: Mechanisms, prevention, and treatment of atrial fibrillation after cardiac surgery, *J Am Coll Cardiol* 51: 793–801, 2008.)

65. **D.** Digoxin is not effective in reducing the risk of developing postoperative atrial fibrillation. In clinical trials, calcium channel blockers, magnesium, statins, polyunsatruated fatty acids, and anti-inflammatory agents such as ketorolac or hydrocortisone have all shown some benefit in reducing the incidence of postoperative atrial fibrillation. However, beta-blockers and amiodarone remain the agents of choice to reduce the risk of postoperative atrial fibrillation.
(See Echahidi N, et al: Mechanisms, prevention, and treatment of atrial fibrillation after cardiac surgery, *J Am Coll Cardiol* 51:793–801, 2008.)

66. **A.** This patient has Brugada syndrome. An ECG taken after a large meal will be positive in nearly 50% of Brugada patients. This patient has recurrent syncope, a class IIa indication for ICD placement. The other options are not indicated in this patient. Beta-blocker therapy does not effectively reduce the risk of sudden death in this patient population.
(See Chen PS, Priori SG: The Brugada syndrome, *J Am Coll Cardiol* 51:1176–1180, 2008.)

67. **C.** Quinidine inhibits the I_{to} channel and has been shown to be an effective treatment for Brugada syndrome. Studies have shown that it prevents the induction of ventricular fibrillation in Brugada patients and may decrease spontaneous arrhythmias in this syndrome. Isoproterenol increases the calcium current and also is effective at suppressing ventricular fibrillation in these patients. However, it is administered intravenously and therefore is not useful as daily therapy.
(See Chen PS, Priori SG: The Brugada syndrome, *J Am Coll Cardiol* 51:1176–1180, 2008.)

68. **False.** B-type natriuretic peptide levels are lower in patients with obesity, but B-type natriuretic peptide levels are still a reliable marker for CHF in obese patients.
(See Ashrafian H, et al: Effects of bariatric surgery on cardiovascular function, *Circulation* 118:2091–2102, 2008; and Horwich TB, et al: B-type natriuretic peptide levels in obese patients with advanced heart failure, *J Am Coll Cardiol* 47:85–90, 2006.)

69. **E.** All of the above are true. A meta-analysis reported that 61% of bariatric surgery patients had an improvement in hypertension, 70% had an improvement in hyperlipidemia, and resolution or improvement of diabetes was seen in 86% of patients. These beneficial effects contribute to a decrease in cardiovascular risk. Mortality has been shown to be improved up to 15 years after surgery.
(See Ashrafian H, et al: Effects of bariatric surgery on cardiovascular function, *Circulation* 118:2091–2102, 2008; and Buchwald H, et al: Bariatric surgery: a systematic review and meta-analysis, *JAMA* 292:1724–1737, 2004.)

70. **C.** An indexed prosthetic valve EOA that is considered mild and usually not clinically significant for the aortic position is a value of >0.85 cm^2/m^2. Moderate patient–prosthesis mismatch is considered an indexed EOA of <0.85 cm^2/m^2. Severe patient–prosthesis mismatch is generally considered at a value of <0.65 cm^2/m^2. The prevalence of severe patient–prosthesis mismatch ranges from 2% to 10%. Patient–prosthesis mismatch of the aortic valve has been associated with less improvement in symptoms, more adverse cardiac events, and increased mortality. Patient–prosthesis mismatch may be more important in patients with decreased LV function. In addition, it may be more important in younger patients than older patients because younger patients may have higher cardiac output needs and are subjected to the effects of patient–prosthesis mismatch for a much longer time.
(See Pibarot P, Dumesnil JG: Prosthetic heart valves: selection of the optimal prosthesis and long-term management, *Circulation* 119: 1034–1048, 2009.)

71. **B.** This patient received a bare metal stent 1 month ago. He now needs a cholecystectomy, which may need to be done via laparotomy, and the surgeon feels there is increased risk of bleeding. Endothelialization of bare metal stents occurs within weeks of implantation; it is generally felt that thienopyridines can be discontinued after 4–6 weeks of therapy if necessary. However, it is recommended that aspirin be continued perioperatively. In addition, there is data to support the continuation of thienopyridine therapy for 1 year after stent placement; therefore, restarting it postoperatively would also be reasonable. A specific dose of aspirin has not been recommended. Studies demonstrating efficacy of administering heparin and glycoprotein IIb/IIIa inhibitors in the perioperative period to prevent stent thrombosis are not available.
(See Fleisher LA, et al: ACC/AHA 2007 guidelines on perioperative cardiovascular evaluation and care for noncardiac surgery, *Circulation* 116:e418–e499, 2007.)

72. **C.** For patients currently taking statins who are scheduled for noncardiac surgery, statins should be continued (class I, level of evidence: B). The first two options are class IIa indications. Beta-blockers are probably recommended for patients undergoing vascular surgery in whom preoperative assessment identifies CAD (class IIa, level of evidence: B). Beta-blockers are probably recommended for patients in whom preoperative assessment for vascular surgery identifies high cardiac risk, as defined by the presence of more than one clinical risk factor (class IIa, level of evidence: B). The usefulness of intraoperative nitroglycerin as a prophylactic agent to prevent myocardial ischemia and cardiac morbidity is unclear for high-risk patients undergoing noncardiac surgery, particularly those who have required nitrate therapy to control angina (class IIb, level of evidence: C). Finally, it is recommended that beta-blockers be continued in patients undergoing surgery who are receiving beta-blockers to treat angina, symptomatic arrhythmias, hypertension, or other ACC/AHA Class I guideline indications (class I, level of evidence: C).
(See Fleisher LA, et al: ACC/AHA 2007 guidelines on perioperative cardiovascular evaluation and care for noncardiac surgery, *Circulation* 116:e418–e499, 2007; and Fleischmann KE, et al: 2009 ACCF/AHA focused update on perioperative beta blockade incorporated into the ACC/AHA 2007 guidelines on perioperative cardiovascular evaluation and care for noncardiac surgery, *Circulation* 120: e169–e276, 2009.)

73. **B.** This patient's vital signs indicate that he is in cardiogenic shock. In patients with STEMI complicated by cardiogenic shock, administering fibrinolytics increases the patient's risk of mortality compared to primary revascularization. Data from the Should We Emergently Revascularize Occluded Coronaries for Cardiogenic Shock (SHOCK) trial demonstrated that patients with STEMI who have cardiogenic shock and are younger than age 75 years who undergo revascularization by PCI or CABG have improved survival compared to those receiving thrombolysis if the revascularization is performed within 18 hours of shock onset. Therefore, patients with STEMI and cardiogenic shock should immediately be transferred to facilities capable of cardiac catheterization and rapid revascularization (PCI or CABG). This is a class I recommendation in the ACC/AHA guidelines for management of STEMI.
(See Antman EM, et al: ACC/AHA guidelines for the management of patients with ST-elevation myocardial infarction, *J Am Coll Cardiol* 44:671–719, 2004; and Antman EM, et al: Focused update of the ACC/AHA 2004 guidelines for the management of patients with ST-elevation myocardial infarction, *Circulation* 117:296–329, 2008; and Kushner FG, et al: 2009 focused updates: ACC/AHA guidelines for the management of patients with ST-elevation myocardial infarction and ACC/AHA/SCAI guidelines on percutaneous coronary, *Circulation* 120:2271–2306, 2009.)

74. **B.** Door to needle time should be <30 minutes in those selected for fibrinolysis. In those selected for PCI, door to balloon time should be <90 minutes. These times reflect the longest acceptable time, and the goal should be to initiate reperfusion therapy as soon as possible.
(See Antman EM, et al: ACC/AHA guidelines for the management of patients with ST-elevation myocardial infarction, *J Am Coll Cardiol* 44:671–719, 2004; and Antman EM, et al: Focused update of the ACC/AHA 2004 guidelines for the management of patients with ST-elevation myocardial infarction, *Circulation* 117:296–329, 2008; and Kushner FG, et al: 2009 focused updates: ACC/AHA guidelines for the management of patients with ST-elevation myocardial infarction and ACC/AHA/SCAI guidelines on percutaneous coronary, *Circulation* 120:2271–2306, 2009.)

75. **C.** Administration of I.V. beta-blockers is a class IIa recommendation (level of evidence: B). Prompt administration of oral beta-blocker to STEMI patients without a contraindication, irrespective of concomitant fibrinolytic therapy or performance of primary PCI, is a class I recommendation (level of evidence: A).
(See Antman EM, et al: ACC/AHA guidelines for the management of patients with ST-elevation myocardial infarction, *J Am Coll Cardiol* 44:671–719, 2004; and Antman EM, et al: Focused update of the ACC/AHA 2004 guidelines for the management of patients with ST-elevation myocardial infarction, *Circulation* 117:296–329, 2008; and Kushner FG, et al: 2009 focused updates: ACC/AHA guidelines for the management of patients with ST-elevation myocardial infarction and ACC/AHA/SCAI guidelines on percutaneous coronary, *Circulation* 120:2271–2306, 2009.)

76. **True.** Although most facilities with PCI capability would favor an early invasive strategy, either strategy is acceptable. If the door to balloon time minus the door to needle time is expected to be longer than 60 minutes, it is generally preferred that fibrinolytics be given immediately.
(See Antman EM, et al: ACC/AHA guidelines for the management of patients with ST-elevation myocardial infarction, *J Am Coll Cardiol* 44:671–719, 2004; and Antman EM, et al: Focused update of the ACC/AHA 2004 guidelines for the management of patients with ST-elevation myocardial infarction, *Circulation* 117:296–329, 2008; and Kushner FG, et al: 2009 focused updates: ACC/AHA guidelines for the management of patients with ST-elevation myocardial infarction and ACC/AHA/SCAI guidelines on percutaneous coronary, *Circulation* 120:2271–2306, 2009.)

77. **C.** All of the other answers are relative contra-indications to fibrinolysis. The other absolute contraindications to fibrinolysis include any prior intracranial hemorrhage, known malignant intracranial neoplasm (primary or metastatic), ischemic stroke within 3 months except acute ischemic stroke within 3 hours, suspected aortic dissection, active bleeding or bleeding diathesis (excluding menses), and significant closed-head or facial trauma within 3 months. The other relative contraindications to fibrinolysis include history of chronic severe poorly controlled hypertension, severe uncontrolled hypertension on presentation (systolic BP > 180 mm Hg or diastolic BP > 110 mm Hg), history of prior ischemic stroke > 3 months, dementia, or known intracranial pathology not covered in contraindications, traumatic or prolonged (>10 minutes) CPR, and noncompressible vascular puncture. Relative contraindications for streptokinase/anistreplase include prior exposure (>5 days ago) or prior allergic reaction to these agents, and current use of anticoagulants; the higher the INR, the higher the risk of bleeding.
(See Antman EM, et al: ACC/AHA guidelines for the management of patients with ST-elevation myocardial infarction, *J Am Coll Cardiol* 44:671–719, 2004; and Antman EM, et al: Focused update of the ACC/AHA 2004 guidelines for the management of patients with ST-elevation myocardial infarction, *Circulation* 117:296–329, 2008; and Kushner FG, et al: 2009 focused updates: ACC/AHA guidelines for the management of patients with ST-elevation myocardial infarction and ACC/AHA/SCAI guidelines on percutaneous coronary, *Circulation* 120:2271–2306, 2009.)

78. **B.** PCI after fibrinolysis is a class IIa indication in patients with ejection fraction <40%, CHF, or serious ventricular arrhythmia. This ventricular arrhythmia may be due to ongoing ischemia; therefore, ICD implantation would be premature. Reperfusion arrhythmias usually occur in the first 24 hours of fibrinolysis and are typically NSVT or an accelerated idioventricular rhythm. Routine PCI after fibrinolytic therapy is a class IIb indication.
(See Antman EM, et al: ACC/AHA guidelines for the management of patients with ST-elevation myocardial infarction, *J Am Coll Cardiol* 44:671–719, 2004; and Antman EM, et al: Focused update of the ACC/AHA 2004 guidelines for the management of patients with ST-elevation myocardial infarction, *Circulation* 117:296–329, 2008; and Kushner FG, et al: 2009 focused updates: ACC/AHA guidelines for the management of patients with ST-elevation myocardial infarction and ACC/AHA/SCAI guidelines on percutaneous coronary, *Circulation* 120:2271–2306, 2009.)

79. **C.** Immediate PCI is indicated in patients who have persistent chest pain, absence of resolution of the ST-segment elevation (at least 50%), or hemodynamic or electrical instability. Clopidogrel should be administered and continued for at least 1 year, but the most important step in this patent's management is immediate coronary angiography and PCI.
(See Antman EM, et al: ACC/AHA guidelines for the management of patients with ST-elevation myocardial infarction, *J Am Coll Cardiol* 44:671–719, 2004; and Antman EM, et al: Focused update of the ACC/AHA 2004 guidelines for the management of patients with ST-elevation myocardial infarction, *Circulation* 117:296–329, 2008; and Kushner FG, et al: 2009 focused updates: ACC/AHA guidelines for the management of patients with ST-elevation myocardial infarction and ACC/AHA/SCAI guidelines on percutaneous coronary, *Circulation* 120:2271–2306, 2009.)

80. **C.** This patient has hypotension and is at risk of clinical deterioration if given I.V. metoprolol. All the other medications are indicated as the patient is being transferred to the cardiac catheterization suite. However, patient transfer should not be delayed to administer medications.
(See Antman EM, et al: ACC/AHA guidelines for the management of patients with ST-elevation myocardial infarction, *J Am Coll Cardiol* 44:671–719, 2004: and Antman EM, et al: Focused update of the ACC/AHA 2004 guidelines for the management of patients with ST-elevation myocardial infarction, *Circulation* 117:296–329, 2008; and Kushner FG, et al: 2009 focused updates: ACC/AHA guidelines for the management of patients with ST-elevation myocardial infarction and ACC/AHA/SCAI guidelines on percutaneous coronary, *Circulation* 120:2271–2306, 2009.)

81. **B.** In post-STEMI patients with LV thrombus noted on an imaging study, warfarin should be prescribed for at least 3 months (class I recommendation, level of evidence: B) and indefinitely in patients without an increased risk of bleeding (class I, level of evidence: C). In addition, it is reasonable to administer warfarin to post-STEMI patients with LV dysfunction and extensive regional wall-motion abnormalities (class IIa, level of evidence: A). ICD placement would only be indicated in this scenario if the patient had ventricular fibrillation or hemodynamically significant sustained VT > 48 hours after STEMI that was not due to transient or reversible ischemia or reinfarction (class I, level of evidence: A). EP study with possible ICD placement is indicated in STEMI patients with an ejection fraction of 31% to 40% (measured at least 1 month postinfarction) who have evidence of electrical instability (e.g., NSVT) (class I, level of evidence: B). There is no indication for NSAID therapy in this patient. In pericarditis after STEMI, NSAIDs may be considered for short-term pain relief but should not be used for extended periods because of their effect on platelet function, a possible association with scar thinning, and infarct expansion (class IIb, level of evidence: B).

(See Antman EM, et al: ACC/AHA guidelines for the management of patients with ST-elevation myocardial infarction, *J Am Coll Cardiol* 44:671–719, 2004; and Antman EM, et al: Focused update of the ACC/AHA 2004 guidelines for the management of patients with ST-elevation myocardial infarction, *Circulation* 117:296–329, 2008; and Kushner FG, et al: 2009 focused updates: ACC/AHA guidelines for the management of patients with ST-elevation myocardial infarction and ACC/AHA/SCAI guidelines on percutaneous coronary, *Circulation* 120:2271–2306, 2009.)

82. **C.** The patient has developed postinfarct pericarditis. There are no clinical signs of tamponade and therefore no current need for pericardiocentesis. High-dose aspirin is a class I indication in this scenario. If aspirin is not successful in controlling her pain, colchicine at 0.6 mg b.i.d. (class IIa, level of evidence: B) or acetaminophen 500 mg orally every 6 hours (class IIa, level of evidence: C) would be the next best choices. Ibuprofen blocks the antiplatelet effect of aspirin and can cause infarct expansion and scar thinning; therefore, it is considered contraindicated (class III, level of evidence: B). Steroids can be used as a last resort in patients with pericarditis refractory to aspirin or NSAIDs, although their use may increase a patient's risk of scar thinning and myocardial rupture.

(See Antman EM, et al: ACC/AHA guidelines for the management of patients with ST-elevation myocardial infarction, *J Am Coll Cardiol* 44:671–719, 2004; and Antman EM, et al: Focused update of the ACC/AHA 2004 guidelines for the management of patients with ST-elevation myocardial infarction, *Circulation* 117:296–329, 2008; and Kushner FG, et al: 2009 focused updates: ACC/AHA guidelines for the management of patients with ST-elevation myocardial infarction and ACC/AHA/SCAI guidelines on percutaneous coronary, *Circulation* 120:2271–2306, 2009.)

83. **C.** Choice A reflects appropriate treatment of sustained polymorphic VT. Choice B is a class IIb indication in this setting, whereas choice C is a class I recommendation. The patient should be sedated before cardioversion. The other class I recommendation in this setting would be amiodarone administration by bolus or infusion, which is not given as an option. Cardiac catheterization would not be the appropriate initial management but may be indicated after the patient's VT is terminated if significant recurrent ischemia or reinfarction is evident.

(See Antman EM, et al: ACC/AHA guidelines for the management of patients with ST-elevation myocardial infarction, *J Am Coll Cardiol* 44:671–719, 2004; and Antman EM, et al: Focused update of the ACC/AHA 2004 guidelines for the management of patients with ST-elevation myocardial infarction, *Circulation* 117:296–329, 2008; and Kushner FG, et al: 2009 focused updates: ACC/AHA guidelines for the management of patients with ST-elevation myocardial infarction and ACC/AHA/SCAI guidelines on percutaneous coronary, *Circulation* 120:2271–2306, 2009.)

84. **D.** This patient may have an intracranial hemorrhage and should have all anticoagulation and antiplatelet therapy discontinued until evaluation for intracranial hemorrhage is complete. After stopping the heparin and aspirin, the patient should undergo an immediate CT of the brain. If an intracranial hemorrhage is present, consultation with neurology, neurosurgery, or hematology should be obtained as clinically indicated. In addition, cryoprecipitate, FFP, protamine, and platelets should be given as clinically appropriate. The above are class I indications. It is also reasonable to control BP and glucose levels and try to reduce ICP by mannitol administration or intubation and hyperventilation (class IIa recommendations).
(See Antman EM, et al: ACC/AHA guidelines for the management of patients with ST-elevation myocardial infarction, *J Am Coll Cardiol* 44:671–719, 2004; and Antman EM, et al: Focused update of the ACC/AHA 2004 guidelines for the management of patients with ST-elevation myocardial infarction, *Circulation* 117:296–329, 2008; and Kushner FG, et al: 2009 focused updates: ACC/AHA guidelines for the management of patients with ST-elevation myocardial infarction and ACC/AHA/SCAI guidelines on percutaneous coronary, *Circulation* 120:2271–2306, 2009.)

85. **A.** The use of I.V., topical, or oral nitrates is useful beyond 48 hours of STEMI for treatment of recurrent angina or persistent CHF as long as nitrate use does not interfere with the use of beta-blockers or ACE inhibitors (class I, level of evidence: B). All of the other answers are class III recommendations. I.V. enalapril should not be used within the first 24 hours of a STEMI secondary to the risk of hypotension. The only exception may be refractory hypertension. Antiarrhythmics should not be routinely given to suppress PVCs, couplets, NSVT, or runs of accelerated idioventricular rhythm. Antioxidant vitamins such as vitamin E and C should not be prescribed to patients with STEMI at discharge to prevent cardiovascular disease.
(See Antman EM, et al: ACC/AHA guidelines for the management of patients with ST-elevation myocardial infarction, *J Am Coll Cardiol* 44:671–719, 2004; and Antman EM, et al: Focused update of the ACC/AHA 2004 guidelines for the management of patients with ST-elevation myocardial infarction, *Circulation* 117:296–329, 2008; and Kushner FG, et al: 2009 focused updates: ACC/AHA guidelines for the management of patients with ST-elevation myocardial infarction and ACC/AHA/SCAI guidelines on percutaneous coronary, *Circulation* 120:2271–2306, 2009.)

86. **E.** This diabetic patient has significant three-vessel disease with depressed LV function. She will benefit from surgical revascularization. However, she had clinical evidence of RV dysfunction on presentation, requiring fluid administration. In addition, all of her antihypertensive medications were held. If she remains free of signs and symptoms of ischemia, she should undergo CABG in approximately 4 weeks to allow recovery of RV contractility.
(See Antman EM, et al: ACC/AHA guidelines for the management of patients with ST-elevation myocardial infarction, *J Am Coll Cardiol* 44:671–719, 2004; and Antman EM, et al: Focused update of the ACC/AHA 2004 guidelines for the management of patients with ST-elevation myocardial infarction, *Circulation* 117:296–329, 2008; and Kushner FG, et al: 2009 focused updates: ACC/AHA guidelines for the management of patients with ST-elevation myocardial infarction and ACC/AHA/SCAI guidelines on percutaneous coronary, *Circulation* 120:2271–2306, 2009.)

87. **D.** This patient presents with stable angina that occurs in a predictable pattern. Stress testing is preferred over coronary angiography in this setting. One may consider performing coronary angiography in the absence of stress testing in a patient with Canadian Cardiovascular Society class III or IV chronic stable angina despite medical therapy (class I, level of evidence: B). Exercise stress ECG would not be the test of choice due to the underlying LBBB. Imaging is necessary, and adenosine myocardial perfusion imaging is preferred to echocardiographic imaging. The LBBB causes abnormal septal motion, which often limits echocardiographic wall-motion interpretation, especially during peak images when the patient is tachycardic.
(See Gibbons RJ, et al: ACC/AHA/ACP-ASIM guidelines for the management of patients with chronic stable angina, *J Am Coll Cardiol* 33:2092–2197, 1999.)

88. **C.** Beta-blockers should not be given to patients in cardiogenic shock or to those at increased risk of developing cardiogenic shock. Risk factors for cardiogenic shock include age > 70 years, systolic BP <120 mm Hg, heart rate > 110 or < 60 bpm, and increased time since onset of symptoms of unstable angina/NSTEMI. The greater the number of risk factors, the higher the risk of cardiogenic shock. All of the other options have a class IA indication in unstable angina/NSTEMI. The patient has a history of GI bleeding, but the question does not state that this is a current or recent problem. Therefore, either UFH or enoxaparin could be used. However, one may choose UFH over enoxaparin in this instance because of the prior history of peptic ulcer disease.
(See Anderson JL, et al: ACC/AHA 2007 guidelines for the management of patients with unstable angina/non–ST-elevation myocardial infarction, *Circulation* 116:e148–e304, 2007.)

89. **D.** Each of the four medications has established efficacy in an early invasive strategy and is given a class I recommendation. However, in a conservative strategy, only the use of UFH, enoxaparin, or fondaparinux is recommended. Bivalirudin only has established efficacy in an early invasive strategy for unstable angina/NSTEMI. In a patient with an increased risk of bleeding, in whom conservative management is planned, fondaparinux is the anticoagulant of choice (class I, level of evidence: B).
(See Anderson JL, et al: ACC/AHA 2007 guidelines for the management of patients with unstable angina/non–ST-elevation myocardial infarction, *Circulation* 116:e148–e304, 2007.)

90. **E.** In patients managed with a conservative strategy, enoxaparin and fondaparinux should be continued for the duration of hospitalization, up to 8 days. UFH should be continued for 48 hours (class I, level of evidence: A).
(See Anderson JL, et al: ACC/AHA 2007 guidelines for the management of patients with unstable angina/non–ST-elevation myocardial infarction, *Circulation* 116:e148–e304, 2007.)

91. **D.** This represents the ideal choice, although individual patient characteristics and bleeding risk may alter the decision to treat with all three agents. Patients that require therapy with aspirin, clopidogrel, and warfarin should have a slightly lower goal INR of 2–2.5 while on all three agents.
(See Anderson JL, et al: ACC/AHA 2007 guidelines for the management of patients with unstable angina/non–ST-elevation myocardial infarction, *Circulation* 116:e148–e304, 2007.)

92. **C.** Fondaparinux is a factor Xa inhibitor that suppresses thrombin formation. In the Organization for the Assessment of Ischemic Strategies trials (OASIS-5 and OASIS-6), it was associated with an increased risk of catheter-associated thrombosis. Therefore, it is currently recommended that fondaparinux be given in conjunction with UFH in an early invasive strategy. Treatment with fondaparinux alone is preferred for those patients with an increased bleeding risk who are managed conservatively.
(See Anderson JL, et al: ACC/AHA 2007 guidelines for the management of patients with unstable angina/non–ST-elevation myocardial infarction, *Circulation* 116:e148–e304, 2007.)

93. **D.** All of the other answers are true. The key to diagnosis of variant angina is documentation of transient ST-segment elevation during an anginal episode. Angina usually occurs at rest but may occur after emotional stress, exercise, hyperventilation, or exposure to cold. The discomfort spontaneously resolves or responds to nitroglycerin. Prolonged vasospasm can cause AV block, MI, VT, or sudden death. ST-segment elevation can be documented on Holter or event ECG monitoring or during treadmill testing performed in the morning. Coronary angiography with or without pharmacologic stimulation may be useful in establishing the diagnosis. Nitrates and calcium antagonists are used to treat this disorder. Patients should stop smoking. Prognosis with treatment is usually good when the coronary arteries are normal or near normal. Prognosis is worse if CAD is present.
(See Anderson JL, et al: ACC/AHA 2007 guidelines for the management of patients with unstable angina/non–ST-elevation myocardial infarction, *Circulation* 116:e148–e304, 2007.)

94. **D.** The patient presents with functional class II symptoms. Her mitral valve area is within the mild range. Her RV systolic pressure is elevated, in the range often seen with moderate mitral stenosis but may be elevated for other reasons, such as her obesity or obstructive sleep apnea. In addition, it is difficult to determine if she is dyspneic secondary to mitral stenosis or from obesity and deconditioning. Therefore, hemodynamic measurements obtained during exercise testing are useful to determine if mitral stenosis is responsible for, or contributing to, the patient's symptoms (class I, level of evidence: C). With exertion, if the patient's PA systolic pressure is >60 mm Hg, or mean transvalvular gradient is >15 mm Hg, or PAWP is >25 mm Hg, the patient likely has symptoms from mitral stenosis and may benefit from percutaneous mitral balloon valvotomy. A TEE is indicated to evaluate the morphology and hemodynamics of the mitral valve if the data obtained from the TTE is suboptimal. TEE is also indicated to evaluate for left atrial thrombus and to assess the severity of mitral regurgitation before balloon valvotomy. A right heart catheterization would allow hemodynamic assessment, but it is invasive and it is not necessary unless hemodynamic assessment by Doppler echocardiography is inadequate (class I, level of evidence: C). Percutaneous mitral balloon valvotomy or mitral valve replacement is premature in this patient without further correlation of symptoms to the valvular disease.
(See Bonow RO, et al: 2008 Focused update incorporated into the ACC/AHA 2006 guidelines for the management of patients with valvular heart disease, *Circulation* 118:e523–e661, 2008.)

95. **E.** This patient has evidence of moderate mitral stenosis with moderate LAE. His symptoms are consistent with a TIA involving his left cerebral hemisphere in the distribution of the left MCA. This most likely was an embolic event occurring from the left atrium. Anticoagulation is recommended in patients with mitral stenosis and an embolic event regardless of whether the patient is in sinus rhythm or atrial fibrillation (class I, level of evidence: B). Anticoagulation is also recommended in patients with mitral stenosis and any history of atrial fibrillation or in those with left atrial thrombus (class I, level of evidence: B). All of the other options are inadquate in this patient.
(See Bonow RO, et al: 2008 Focused update incorporated into the ACC/AHA 2006 guidelines for the management of patients with valvular heart disease, *Circulation* 118:e523–e661, 2008.)

96. **C.** In patients with mitral valve prolapse and atrial fibrillation, warfarin is recommended for patients with any of the following: hypertension, mitral regurgitation murmur, history of CHF, or age older than 65 years (class I, level of evidence: C). Aspirin at 75–325 mg is recommended for those patients with mitral valve prolapse and atrial fibrillation who are younger than age 65 years with no history of mitral regurgitation, hypertension, or heart failure (class I, level of evidence: C). Aspirin is recommended in patients with mitral valve prolapse who have had a TIA (class I, level of evidence: C). If a patient with mitral valve prolapse has a stroke and mitral regurgitation, atrial fibrillation, or left atrial thrombus is present, warfarin is recommended (class I, level of evidence: C).
(See Bonow RO, et al: 2008 Focused update incorporated into the ACC/AHA 2006 guidelines for the management of patients with valvular heart disease, *Circulation* 118:e523–e661, 2008.)

97. **D.** Bidirectional VT is characterized by a beat-to-beat alternans in the QRS frontal plane axis and is associated with digoxin toxicity. Paroxysmal atrial tachycardia with varying degrees of AV block and ventricular bigeminy are also commonly associated with digoxin toxicity.
(See Zipes DP, et al: ACC/AHA/ESC 2006 guidelines for management of patients with ventricular arrhythmias and the prevention of sudden cardiac death, *Circulation* 114:e385–e484, 2006.)

98. **D.** Acute and long-term pacing is recommended for patients with torsades de pointes due to heart block and symptomatic bradycardia (class I, level of evidence: A) and is reasonable in those patients with pause-dependent torsades de pointes (class IIa, level of evidence: B). Temporary transvenous pacing and beta-blocker therapy in combination is recommended for patients who have torsades de pointes and sinus bradycardia (class IIa, level of evidence: C). Magnesium may be useful in patients with torsades de pointes who also have long QT syndrome. Magnesium is unlikely to be helpful in patients with a normal QT interval (class IIa, level of evidence: B). Isoproterenol may be used temporarily to treat torsades de pointes in patients who do not have congenital long QT syndrome (class IIa, level of evidence: B).
(See Zipes DP, et al: ACC/AHA/ESC 2006 guidelines for management of patients with ventricular arrhythmias and the prevention of sudden cardiac death, *Circulation* 114:e385–e484, 2006.)

99. **C.** All of the other options are considered major risk factors for sudden cardiac death in HCM. The other major risk factors include cardiac arrest secondary to ventricular fibrillation, spontaneous sustained VT, family history of premature sudden death, and abnormal exercise BP. Possible risk factors that may be important in individual patients include atrial fibrillation, myocardial ischemia, LV outflow obstruction, and intense (competitive) physical exertion. The above risk factors were categorized in this manner in a consensus document on HCM from the American College of Cardiology and the European Society of Cardiology. ICD implantation can be effective for primary prevention of sudden cardiac death in HCM patients who have one or more major risk factors and are receiving chronic optimal medical therapy. Patients should have a reasonable expectation of survival with good functional status for >1 year (class IIa, level of evidence: C).
(See Zipes DP, et al: ACC/AHA/ESC 2006 guidelines for management of patients with ventricular arrhythmias and the prevention of sudden cardiac death, *Circulation* 114:e385–e484, 2006.)

100. **D.** In patients with atrial fibrillation, administration of I.V. beta-blockers or nondihydropyridine calcium channel blockers is indicated in the acute setting, in the absence of heart failure or preexcitation, to achieve rate control. However, the patient in the question has clinical signs and symptoms of heart failure; therefore, esmolol and diltiazem should not be used. Even though the patient is in heart failure, there is no evidence from the information provided in the question that she is hemodynamically unstable; therefore, performing immediate cardioversion is not indicated. Nonetheless, if an urgent cardioversion is deemed necessary, administration of a bolus of I.V. heparin and then a drip is indicated. This patient is in heart failure (and preexcitation is absent on the ECG); therefore, for rate control, I.V. amiodarone or digoxin is recommended. Caution with I.V. digoxin would be indicated in this patient because she has chronic kidney disease. Giving a bolus of amiodarone may precipitate hypotension. Giving the bolus slowly over approximately 20 minutes may diminish the likelihood of this complication. I.V. amiodarone is indicated for achieving rate control in patients with heart failure or in critically ill patients with hypotension (such as patients with sepsis).
(See Fuster V, et al: ACC/AHA/ESC 2006 guidelines for the management of patients with atrial fibrillation, *Circulation* 114:e257–e354.)

INDEX